EXPERIMENTAL FOODS LABORATORY MANUAL

Sixth Edition

by Margaret McWilliams, Ph.D., R.D.

Professor Emeritus
California State University, Los Angeles

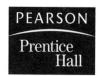

PEARSON
Prentice
Hall

Upper Saddle River, New Jersey 07458

Executive Editor: Vernon R. Anthony
Senior Marketing Coordinator: Elizabeth Farrell
Marketing Assistant: Les Roberts
Editorial Assistant: Beth Dyke
Associate Editor: Linda Cupp
Director of Manufacturing and Production: Bruce Johnson
Managing Editor: Mary Carnis
Production Liaison: Janice Stangel
Senior Marketing Manager: Ryan DeGrote
Production Management: Pine Tree Composition, Inc.
Production Editor: Bruce Hobart
Manufacturing Manager: Ilene Sanford
Manufacturing Buyer: Cathleen Petersen
Creative Director: Cheryl Asherman
Cover Design Coordinator: Mary Siener
Interior Design: Pine Tree Composition, Inc.
Printer/Binder: Banta Book Group
Cover Designer: Allen Gold
Cover Printer: Phoenix Color

Pearson Prentice Hall™ is a trademark of Pearson Education, Inc.
Pearson® is a registered trademark of Pearson plc
Prentice Hall® is a registered trademark of Pearson Education, Inc.

Pearson Education LTD
Pearson Education Australia PTY, Limited
Pearson Education Singapore, Pte.Ltd
Pearson Education North Asia Ltd
Pearson Education Canada, Ltd

Pearson Educación de Mexico, S.A. de C.V.
Pearson Education—Japan
Pearson Education Malaysia, Pte. Ltd
Pearson Education, Upper Saddle River, New Jersey

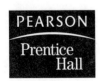

10 9 8 7 6 5 4 3 2 1
ISBN 0-13-039483-1

EXPERIMENTAL FOODS LABORATORY MANUAL

Books by the Author

Food around the World: A Cultural Perspective
(with Holly Heller)
Prentice Hall, 2003

Fundamentals of Meal Management, 1st ed.
Prentice Hall, 2005

Foods: Experimental Perspectives, 5th ed.
Prentice Hall, 2005

Experimental Foods Laboratory Manual, 5th ed.
Plycon Press, 2000

Food Fundamentals, 7th ed.
Plycon Press, 1998

Illustrated Guide to Food Preparation, 8th ed.
Plycon Press, 1998

Nutrition for the Growing Years, 5th ed.
Plycon Press, 1993

Fundamentals of Meal Management, 3rd ed.
Plycon Press, 1997

Meatless Cookbook
Plycon Press, 1974

Living Nutrition, 4th ed.
(with Fredrick Stare, Ph.D., M.D.)
Macmillan, 1984

Nutrition for Good Health, 2nd ed.
Stickley, 1982

Modern Food Preservation
(with Harriett Paine)
Plycon Press, 1977

Understanding Food
(with Lendal Kotschevar)
Wiley, 1969

Food For You, 2nd ed.
(with Linda Davis)
Ginn, 1976

World of Nutrition
(with Holly Heller)
Ginn, 1988

Contents

Index of Charts

Preface

This laboratory manual is designed to help students illustrate many of the principles of food science. Careful preparation and evaluation of the samples in each experiment develop important laboratory skills. Analysis of the results promotes understanding of the principles demonstrated in each experiment, and learning is reinforced by written responses to the study questions at the end of each experiment.

Experiments for studying crystallization, starch, vegetables and fruits, fats and oils, dairy products, flesh foods, eggs, leavening agents, baked products, and food preservation are presented. Objectives, procedures, evaluation techniques and charts, and study questions are provided for each experiment.

Appendix A will help students become familiar with laboratory techniques used in preparing samples and with operating some of the objective testing equipment. Students can refer to this information as questions arise in the laboratory. Appendices B, C, D, E, and F will be useful to students as they proceed through the experiments.

All students in the laboratory contribute to the success of each experiment because accurate preparation of each sample is critical to illustrating exactly what the result of the variation should be. Errors in quantities of ingredients and/or in their preparation present incorrect information on the display tables where samples are being examined and evaluated. When students prepare products accurately, samples will clearly illustrate the effects of each variation, and learning is facilitated.

It is important to realize that some samples will seem like failures if they have been prepared correctly. "Planned failures" are included in these experiments because students need to observe the effects of varying ingredients and preparation techniques.

The charts at the end of each experiment are designed to help students organize their evaluation comments while still in the laboratory. All samples need to be labeled accurately before being placed in the designated position on the display table (with serving silverware, if needed). When samples are arranged systematically in the same sequence as the charts, evaluation by students can be done efficiently and accurately.

Students will develop the essentials needed for functioning in a research laboratory, consumer service facility, or food service as they carefully work through the range of experiments presented in this book. From this foundation in the food science laboratory, students can make the transition into professional situations that will extend their knowledge and abilities.

Now it is time to go into the lab and begin the experiments!

Margaret McWilliams
Redondo Beach, California

EXPERIMENTAL FOODS LABORATORY MANUAL

1
Crystallization

Controlled crystal formation is the key to obtaining a desirable texture in crystalline candies and frozen desserts. In the case of sugar crystallization, the results are influenced by: (1) the ingredients; (2) the rate of cooking; (3) the final concentration of sugar; and (4) the conditions during cooling. If the concentration of sugar is very high (indicated generally by temperatures above 121°C) when cooking ceases, the formation of sugar crystals is inhibited by the very viscous nature of the solution, and an amorphous candy will be the result. However, it is the crystalline candies resulting when the concentration of sugar is somewhat lower that are of interest in this chapter. The following experiments on crystalline candies illustrate the chemical changes and physical factors influencing the textural characteristics of the finished product.

Frozen desserts provide a different illustration of crystallization, for they contain ice crystals. The size of these ice crystals and their density are

EXPERIMENT 1.1—CRYSTALLINE CANDIES
OBJECTIVES

Upon completion of the experiment, you will be able to:

1. Explain the interrelationship of the boiling temperature of a sugar solution and the firmness of the resulting candy.
2. Discuss the factors influencing the firmness of a crystalline candy.
3. Identify the factors influencing the texture of a crystalline candy and explain the action of each.
4. Define a super-saturated solution and explain its significance in making high-quality crystalline candies.
5. Explain why the rate of cooking influences the firmness and texture of crystalline candies.

BASIC FORMULA—FONDANT

200 g   Sugar
118 ml   Water

Place the sugar and water in a 1-quart heavy saucepan on the range. Position a ring stand and a suspended laboratory thermometer so that the bulb of the thermometer is completely immersed in the sugar solution, but not touching the bottom of the pan. Unless preparing the slow-cooking samples (1a, 1c, and 1e), begin heating at the highest setting, but reduce the heat as necessary to prevent the fondant from boiling over. Stir with a wooden spoon while bringing to a boil. Continue stirring slowly until just before reaching the final temperature of 113°C (for all samples except 2a and 2b). The cooking time required should be about 10 minutes. When the thermometer reaches 113°C, remove the fondant from the range, leaving the thermometer suspended in a position so that it can be read without moving it. Avoid disturbing the fondant at all until the temperature drops to 40°C. Then beat vigorously with a wooden spoon until the fondant loses its gloss and is about to set (20 minutes maximum on variations). If necessary, knead until smooth. Evaluate half the fondant. Wrap the remaining half of the fondant tightly in aluminum foil for evaluation during the next period.

---

important factors in determining the texture of frozen products. The ingredient formulation, the rate of freezing, and the amount of agitation are all factors influencing the texture of these products. The experiments on ice cream in this chapter demonstrate the influence of these various factors.

1. **Rate of cooking.** (Although precise time control is not possible in a classroom situation, attempt to regulate the rate of heating as accurately as possible.)

   a. *Slow rate (20 minutes)*—Use the basic formula ingredients. Bring the candy to a boil and continue to boil slowly so that the entire cooking period requires about 20 minutes to reach 113°C.

   b. *Fast rate (10 minutes)*—Prepare the basic formula. This sample is the control.

   c. *Slow rate + cream of tartar*—Add 0.5 g cream of tartar to the basic formula and follow the cooking instructions in 1a.

   d. *Fast rate + cream of tartar*—Prepare the basic formula, but add 0.5 g cream of tartar before beginning to cook the solution.

   e. *Slow rate + corn syrup*—Add 15 ml corn syrup to the basic formula; follow the cooking instructions in 1a.

   f. *Fast rate + corn syrup*—Prepare the basic formula, but add 15 ml corn syrup to the solution before cooking.

2. **Final temperature**

   a. *111°C*—Prepare the basic formula, but cook to a final temperature of only 111°C.

   b. *115°C*—Prepare the basic formula, but cook to a final temperature of 115°C.

3. **Varying ingredients**

   a. *Butter at beginning*—Prepare the basic formula, but add 14 g butter before cooking the solution.

   b. *Butter after cooking*—Prepare the basic formula, but add 14 g butter when the candy is removed from the range. Let the butter melt on the surface without stirring it at all.

   c. *Butter + cream of tartar*—Prepare the basic formula, but add 0.5 g cream of tartar at the beginning (before cooking), and add 14 g butter at the end of the cooking period (without stirring).

   d. *Lemon juice (5 ml)*—Prepare the basic formula, but add 5 ml strained lemon juice before beginning to cook.

   e. *Lemon juice (15 ml)*—Prepare the basic formula, but add 15 ml strained lemon juice before beginning to cook.

   f. *Corn syrup (30 ml)*—Prepare the basic formula, but add 30 ml of corn syrup before beginning to cook.

   g. *Corn syrup (60 ml)*—Prepare the basic formula, but add 60 ml corn syrup before beginning to cook.

   h. *Cream of tartar (1.5 g)*—Prepare the basic formula, but add 1.5 g cream of tartar before beginning to cook.

   i. *Distilled water*—Prepare the basic formula, but use distilled water in place of tap water.

   j. *Cream*—Prepare the basic formula, but use cream in place of tap water.

BASIC FORMULA—FUDGE

200 g	Sugar
118 ml	Cream (half and half)
28 g	Chocolate, unsweetened
14 g	Butter

Place sugar, cream, and chocolate in a 1-qt heavy saucepan. Position it on the range with a ring stand adjacent so it can support a thermometer with its bulb immersed in the candy, but not touching the bottom of the pan. Heat slowly at first while stirring with a wooden spoon. After the chocolate has melted, increase the rate of heating to boil the mixture rapidly. Boil to a final temperature of 112°C. Remove from the heat, but leave the thermometer in the candy so it can be read without moving it. Immediately add the butter without stirring. Let cool undisturbed until temperature drops to 40°C. Then beat vigorously with a wooden spoon until the fudge loses its gloss and appears to be ready to set (or a maximum of 20 minutes on variations). Knead, if necessary. Use half for evaluating the fresh product. Wrap half the fudge in aluminum foil for evaluation at the next laboratory period.

4. **Ingredient variations**

   a. *Water*—Prepare the basic fudge formula, but substitute water for the cream.

   b. *Cream*—Prepare the basic fudge formula. This is the control.

   c. *Cream of tartar*—Prepare the basic fudge formula, but add 0.5 g cream of tartar before beginning to cook the fudge.

   d. *Cream of tartar and corn syrup*—Prepare the basic fudge formula, but add 0.5 g cream of tartar and 30 ml corn syrup before beginning to cook the fudge.

5. **Temperature and ingredient variations**

   a. *114°C, basic with water*—Prepare the basic fudge formula, but use water in place of cream and boil to a final temperature of 114°C.

   b. *114°C, basic formula*—Prepare the basic fudge formula, but boil to a final temperature of 114°C.

   c. *114°C, cream of tartar*—Prepare the basic fudge formula, but add 0.5 g cream of tartar before beginning to cook the fudge and boil to a final temperature of 114°C.

   d. *114C, cream of tartar, corn syrup*—Prepare the basic fudge formula, but add 0.5 g cream of tartar and 30 ml corn syrup before beginning to cook the fudge. Boil the fudge to a final temperature of 114°C.

6. **Cocoa**

   a. *Cocoa + butter*—Prepare the basic fudge formula, but substitute 22.5 g cocoa and an additional 7 g butter for the chocolate.

   b. *Cocoa + butter, 114°C*—Prepare the basic fudge formula, but substitute 22.5 g cocoa and an additional 7 g butter for the chocolate. Boil this fudge to a final temperature of 114°C.

7. **Temperature of beating**—The following variations are made to demonstrate the importance of supersaturation in relation to texture of the finished product. The basic formula is fudge.

   a. *Beat at 112°C*—Prepare the basic fudge formula, but begin to beat the fudge as soon as it is removed from the heat and continue to beat until firm. Knead.

   b. *Beat at 112°C for 2 minutes*—Prepare the basic fudge formula, but begin to beat as soon as it is removed from the heat and beat for 2 minutes. Stop beating and allow the candy to finish cooling without further disturbance.

   c. *Beat at 80°C*—Prepare the basic fudge formula, but cool undisturbed to 80°C before beginning to beat the fudge. Continue beating according to directions in the basic fudge formula.

   d. *Beat at 60°C*—Prepare the basic fudge formula, but cool undisturbed to 60°C before beginning to beat the fudge. Proceed with beating according to the basic fudge formula.

EVALUATION

Microscope   Place a drop of turpentine on a microscope slide and add a very small grain of the candy. Place a cover slip on top and slide it around to make a very thin layer of the candy crystals. View under the microscope. Under the microscope, compare the size of the crystals in the various treatments in the total experiment.

Penetrometer   Place a 1-inch cube of the product on the penetrometer platform. Use the needle attachment, and release it for 60 seconds. Measure and record the penetration of the samples.

Subjective evaluation   Evaluate each candy for color, flavor, firmness, and texture. Texture is of particular concern and can be evaluated best by rubbing the sample against the roof of the mouth with the aid of the tongue. Make very careful notes about firmness and texture of the samples on the day they are made so that they can be recalled accurately when evaluation is done on the stored samples in the following laboratory period.

STUDY QUESTIONS

1. Describe and explain the effect of the rate of cooking on each of the following fondant variations:

   a. Basic formula

   b. Added cream of tartar

   c. Added corn syrup

2. What effect can be observed as the final temperature of the candy is increased? Is the sugar concentration increased, decreased, or unchanged as the temperature of the boiling candy rises?

3. Which added ingredients influence the firmness of crystalline candies? Explain the effect of each ingredient.

4. What functions does butter perform in fudge?

5. What is the purpose of adding cream of tartar in fondant?

6. Does the temperature at which beating is initiated influence the firmness of fudge? Explain.

7. Does the temperature at which beating is initiated influence the smoothness of fudge? Explain.

8. Write the chemical reaction that occurs when cream of tartar is used in making fondant. Is this the same type of reaction that occurs when lemon juice is added? When corn syrup is added?

9. What is a supersaturated solution? How is it made? Why is it important in sugar cookery?

CHART 1.1   EFFECTS OF VARYING PROCEDURES AND INGREDIENTS ON CRYSTALLINE CANDIES

Treatment	Micro-scope	Pene-trometer	Color	Flavor	Firmness		Texture	
					Fresh	Ripened	Fresh	Ripened
Fondant								
1. Cook rate								
a. Slow, basic								
b. Fast, basic (control)								
c. Slow, cream tartar								
d. Fast, cream tartar								
e. Slow, corn syrup								
f. Fast, corn syrup								
2. Final temperature								
a. 111°C								
b. 115°C								
3. Ingredients								
a. Butter, beginning								
b. Butter, end								
c. Butter, cream tartar								
d. Lemon, 5 ml								
e. Lemon, 15 ml								
f. Corn syrup, 30 ml								
g. Corn syrup, 60 ml								
h. Cream tartar, 1.5 g								
i. Distilled water								
j. Cream								
Fudge								
4. Ingredients								
a. Water								
b. Cream (control)								
c. Cream tartar								
d. Cr. tartar, corn syrup								
5. Temperature								
a. 114°C, water								
b. 114°C, cream								
c. 114°C, cr. tartar								
d. 114°C, cr. tar., corn syr.								
6. Cocoa								
a. Cocoa, butter, 112°C								
b. Cocoa, butter, 114°C								
7. Temp. beating								
a. 112°C								
b. 112°C, 2 min.								
c. 80°C								
d. 60°C								

Name

ADDITIONAL OBSERVATIONS AND NOTES

EXPERIMENT 1.2—VARIABLES INFLUENCING ICE CREAMS
OBJECTIVES

Upon completion of the experiment, you will be able to:

1. Explain the role of fat and protein materials as interfering substances in ice creams.
2. Interpret the effect of varying levels of sugar on the freezing point of ice cream mixtures.
3. Define overrun in ice cream and identify the factors that contribute to it.
4. Identify the factors that influence the texture and mouthfeel of ice creams.

BASIC FORMULA—FRENCH ICE CREAM

24 g	Egg yolk
50 g	Sugar
0.25 g	Salt
118 ml	Milk
8 ml	Vanilla
118 ml	Whipping cream

Beat the egg yolk and blend with sugar, salt, and milk. Heat slowly to 85°C, stirring constantly with a wooden spoon. Add the vanilla and pour into a metal loaf pan. Measure and record the depth of the mixture in the pan. Then place on the bottom of the freezer, being sure the freezer is set on its coldest setting. Freeze for about 30 minutes (until mushy). Beat the whipping cream until just stiff enough to pile. Transfer the freezing mixture from the metal loaf pan to a chilled bowl; beat on the mixer just until smooth. Fold in whipped cream, return to metal pan, and place on the bottom of the freezer. Stir thoroughly every 10 minutes during the first half hour, then at 15-minute intervals the second half hour. Let mixture continue to freeze until firm (probably about 2 more hours). If evaluation cannot be done until the following period, cover the metal pan very tightly with aluminum foil and leave in freezer. Turn freezer setting back to normal at the end of period. Measure the depth of the frozen ice cream and record.

1. **Stabilizers and additives**—The following series includes substances that help stabilize the ice cream and delay its melting when served. All of the substances should be viewed from their role in modifying the texture of the frozen product, too.

   a. *Control*—Prepare the basic formula as written.

   b. *Cornstarch paste*—Prepare the basic formula, but add 8 g (1 tbsp) cornstarch with the sugar-milk mixture and bring the mixture to a boil while stirring constantly.

   c. *Unwhipped cream*—Prepare the basic formula, but add the whipping cream without whipping it.

d. *Gelatin (3 1/2 g)*—Prepare the basic formula, but blend 3 1/2 g (1/2 envelope) of plain gelatin thoroughly with the sugar; chill only until syrupy before folding in whipping cream.

e. *Gelatin (7 g)*—Repeat 1d, but use 7 g gelatin.

f. *Egg white meringue*—Prepare the basic formula, but reserve 25 g of the sugar for use in making a meringue. At the same time when the whipped cream is being prepared for incorporation, in a separate bowl beat 33 g of egg white until foamy and then gradually beat in the 25 g of sugar reserved above. Beat until the peaks just bend over. Fold this meringue into the ice cream at the same time the whipped cream is being added. Mark on the pan the level of the ice cream mixture.

g. *Salad oil*—Prepare the basic formula, but add 15 ml salad oil to the custard mixture.

h. *Chocolate*—Add 28 g of semi-sweet chocolate (chocolate chips or square) to the custard sauce. Be sure all chocolate is melted before chilling begins.

i. *Evaporated milk*—Prepare the basic formula, but use evaporated milk (unreconstituted) in place of the milk in the custard.

j. *Sweetened condensed milk*—Prepare the basic formula, but use sweetened condensed milk in place of the milk and delete the sugar in the custard.

2. **Types and amounts of sweeteners**

a. *Honey*—Prepare the basic formula, but use 59 ml honey in place of the sugar.

b. *Corn syrup*—Prepare the basic formula, but use 30 ml corn syrup and 25 g sugar total for sweetening.

c. *Sucralose*—Prepare the basic formula, but use 6 g sucralose in place of the 50 g sugar.

d. *75 g sugar (1.5 times)*—Prepare the basic formula, but use a total of 75 g sugar.

e. *100 g sugar (2 times)*—Prepare the basic formula, but use a total of 100 g sugar.

f. *150 g sugar (3 times)*—Prepare the basic formula, but use a total of 150 g sugar.

3. **Freezing techniques**—Note time to freeze.

a. *No stirring*—Prepare the basic formula, but stir whipped cream into custard mixture at start of freezing and do not stir again at all.

b. *No stirring after whipped cream folded in*—Follow the basic formula until the whipped cream has been folded into the frozen mush. Do not stir any other time during freezing.

c. *Stir 1 time after whipped cream is in*—Follow the basic formula, but stir freezing mixture only 1 time after the whipped cream has been folded in. This 1 stirring should be done 30 minutes after starting to freeze the product containing the whipped cream.

d. *Stir 2 times after whipped cream is in*—Stir the basic formula mixture only two times after the whipped cream is in. The stirring times should be after 30 minutes and after 45 minutes.

e. *Ice cream freezer*—Prepare the basic formula, but incorporate the whipped cream when the custard mixture has cooled to room temperature. Place in the container of a crank-type freezer. Pack the freezer with a mixture of ¼ c ice cream salt or rock salt to 1 qt chipped ice. Note the total cranking time required to freeze the ice cream.

EVALUATION

Objective assessment   Overrun is of interest because of the relationship to yield and also its influence on mouthfeel. The volumes to be used in the following equation are determined by measuring the amount of water required to fill the loaf pan (used for freezing the ice cream) to the same depth as was measured (1) before freezing and (2) after freezing.

$$\% \text{ overrun} = \frac{\text{volume (frozen)} - \text{volume (unfrozen)}}{\text{volume (unfrozen)}} \times 100$$

Subjective evaluation   Measure the quality of ice cream subjectively by placing the pans containing the ice creams on crushed ice during the subjective evaluation to minimize melting and promote evaluation of structure.

When evaluating stabilizers, it is helpful to let a small amount of the ice cream melt and observe the tendency of the melted mixture to hold the original shape and volume. If possible, position a thermometer bulb in the middle of the ice cream to be melted. Note the temperature at which the ice cream begins to melt.

STUDY QUESTIONS

1. Do any of the ingredients tested as additives or in the original formula influence the freezing temperature of the ice cream? If so, which ingredient(s) and how much?

2. What is the effect of freezing a refrigerator ice cream without stirring?

3. Did the ice creams made in the freezer of the refrigerator freeze more quickly than the cranked ice cream? Why?

4. What would be the effect on the ease of serving if the level of sugar in an ice cream were increased significantly? Why?

5. Describe the sensory qualities that are characteristic of a high quality ice cream.

6. Can various sweeteners and sugars be substituted for sucrose in ice cream? Describe the probable effects of each substitution you suggest.

7. What is overrun? Is it important? Can an ice cream have too much overrun? Can it have too little overrun? Explain.

8. What can be done to improve the texture and mouthfeel of ice creams deemed to need improvement?

CHART 1.2 EVALUATION OF ICE CREAM

Treatment	M.P. temp (°C)	% Overrun	Color	Flavor	Texture	Mouthfeel
1. Stabilizers, additives a. Control						
b. Cornstarch						
c. Unwhipped cream						
d. 3 1/2 g gelatin						
e. 7 g gelatin						
f. Meringue						
g. Salad oil						
h. Chocolate						
i. Evaporated milk						
j. Sweet cond. milk						
2. Sweeteners a. Honey						
b. Corn syrup						
c. Sucralose						
d. 1 1/2 x sugar						
e. 2x sugar						
f. 3x sugar						
3. Freezing techniques a. No stir						
b. No stir after adding whip. cr.						
c. Stir 1x						
d. Stir 2x						
e. Ice cream freezer						

Name

ADDITIONAL OBSERVATIONS AND NOTES

2
Starch

Starch from various sources is used as a thickening agent in a wide range of products. In the home, starch may be the primary thickener in soups, sauces for casseroles and meats (including gravies), sauces for vegetables, some salad dressings, and various desserts, such as dessert soufflés, pie fillings, and puddings. Starch is a significant component of cereals and legumes, too, and accounts for the swelling that takes place in these products as they are cooked.

The process of gelatinization is essential to the achievement of the correct viscosity of starch pastes and the desired characteristics of starch gels. Different starches will contribute varying degrees of thickening power and translucency to starch pastes and gels. Some of them will exhibit thinning with prolonged heating, and some will not form gels. To use the various starches to best advantage, it is necessary to be familiar with the characteristics of each type. These cereal and legume experiments are designed to illustrate the different types of starch products available today and to provide comparisons between cooking time, yields, and cost.

EXPERIMENT 2.1—STARCH PASTES AND GELS
OBJECTIVES

Upon completion of the experiment, you will be able to:

1. Explain the process of gelatinization.
2. Compare the behavior and appearance of the gelatinized starches prepared in this experiment.
3. Define a starch gel and a starch sol.
4. Discuss the factors that influence the viscosity of products that are thickened by starch.

BASIC FORMULA—STARCH PASTE

16 g	Starch
236 ml	Water

Slowly stir water into the starch in a 1-qt heavy aluminum saucepan. Cook over direct heat while stirring to prevent lumping. Heat to boiling unless mixture appears to start to thin. (If mixture starts to thin, immediately note the temperature and stop heating.) If thinning is not apparent, bring to a full boil. Perform a line spread test (see Appendix A and Appendix D). Then the sols in variations 1 and 3 are prepared for further testing by placing each sol in a custard cup, covering tightly, and placing in a shallow pan of ice water to cool. Evaluation is described in the section following the variations.

1. **Varying concentration of various starches**

    a. *Waxy cornstarch, 16 g*—Prepare the basic formula, using waxy cornstarch as the starch.

    b. *Waxy cornstarch, 8 g*—Prepare the basic formula, but use only 8 g waxy cornstarch.

    c. *Cornstarch, 16 g*—Prepare the basic formula, using cornstarch. (This can be used as the control for series 3.)

    d. *Cornstarch, 8 g*—Prepare the basic formula, but use only 8 g cornstarch.

    e. *Rice starch, 16 g*—Prepare the basic formula, using rice starch.

    f. *Rice starch, 8 g*—Prepare the basic formula, but use only 8 g rice starch.

    g. *Quick-cooking tapioca, 16 g*—Prepare the basic formula, using quick-cooking tapioca as the starch.

    h. *Quick-cooking tapioca, 8 g*—Prepare the basic formula, but use only 8 g quick-cooking tapioca.

    i. *Potato starch, 16g*—Prepare the basic formula, using potato starch as the starch.

    j. *Potato starch, 8 g*—Prepare the basic formula, but use only 8 g potato starch.

    k. *Wheat starch, 16 g*—Prepare the basic formula, using wheat starch as the starch.

    l. *Wheat starch, 8 g*—Prepare the basic formula, but use only 8 g wheat starch.

    m. *All purpose flour, 16 g*—Prepare the basic formula, using all purpose flour for the starch.

n. *All purpose flour, 8 g*—Prepare the basic formula, but use only 8 g all purpose flour.

o. *Dextrinized flour, 16 g*—Prepare the basic formula, using dextrinized flour. Dextrinized flour is made by browning (while stirring) all purpose flour in a dry skillet until the flour is a uniform medium-brown color.

2. **Temperature of maximum gelatinization**—Prepare assigned samples as follows. Suspend a thermometer in the pan so that the bulb is covered by the starch mixture, but is not touching the bottom of the pan. Stir while heating the starch sol. Remove enough of the sol when the temperature reaches 70°C to conduct a line spread test. Place a teaspoonful of the sample from the line spread test on a watch glass for later evaluation by the class. Return the rest of the sample to the pan and continue stirring while heating the sol to 80°C. Test in the same manner as for the 70°C sample. Repeat tests at 90°C, 95°C, and when the mixture boils (or at the maximum temperature that can be reached).

a. *Waxy cornstarch*—Prepare double the basic formula, using 32 g waxy cornstarch and 472 ml water.

b. *Cornstarch*—Prepare double the basic formula, using 32 g cornstarch and 472 ml water.

c. *Rice starch*—Prepare double the basic formula, using 32 g rice starch and 472 ml water.

d. *Quick-cooking tapioca*—Prepare double the basic formula, using 32 g quick-cooking tapioca and 472 ml water.

e. *Potato starch*—Prepare double the basic formula, using 32 g potato starch and 472 ml water.

f. *Wheat starch*—Prepare double the basic formula, using 32 g wheat starch and 472 ml water.

g. *All purpose flour*—Prepare double the basic formula, using 32 g all purpose flour and 472 ml water.

h. *Dextrinized flour*—Prepare double the basic formula, using 64 g dextrinized (see 1.o) all purpose flour and 472 ml water.

3. **Effect of acid and sugar**—To illustrate the effect of acid and sugar on gelatinizing starch mixtures, prepare the following variations using cornstarch as the thickening agent.

a. *0 g sugar (control)*—Prepare the basic formula (using cornstarch) or use 1.c as the control.

b. *25 g sugar*—Prepare the basic formula and add 25 g sugar with the cornstarch.

c. *50 g sugar*—Prepare the basic formula and add 50 g sugar with the cornstarch.

d. *30 ml lemon juice*—Prepare the basic formula (use cornstarch), but use 30 ml lemon juice and 206 ml water. Measure the pH.

e. *60 ml lemon juice*—Prepare the basic formula (use cornstarch), but use 60 ml lemon juice and 176 ml water. Measure the pH.

f. *25 g sugar, 30 ml lemon juice*—Prepare the basic formula (use cornstarch), but add 25 g sugar with the cornstarch and use 30 ml lemon juice and 206 ml water.

4. **Gelatinization of cereals and legumes**—Prepare the following products according to package directions. Use 60 ml (1/4 c) of the cereal assigned and the amount of water specified in the directions on the package.

a. *Minute rice*

b. *Parboiled rice*

c. *Polished rice (long grain)*

d. *Polished rice (short grain)*

e. *Instant oatmeal*

f. *Quick oatmeal*

g. *Regular oatmeal*

h. *Navy beans*(60 ml dry beans that have been soaked overnight)

EVALUATION

Objective testing
Group 1 variations

- *Line spread* (30 seconds) on both the hot paste and the chilled sample (if product is still a paste). See Appendix A for instructions.
- *Penetrometer* on all products that gel. All samples should be tested with the same cone for the same length of time (determined when the first sample is tested). See Appendix A for instructions.
- *Percent sag* on all products that gel. See Appendix A for instructions.

Group 2 variations

- *Line spread* on hot paste at 70°C, 80°C, 90°C, 95°C, and boiling. See Appendix A for instructions.

Group 3 variations

- *Line spread* on both the hot paste and chilled sample if it still is a paste. See Appendix A for instructions.
- *Penetrometer* on both the hot paste and the chilled sample if product still is a paste. See Appendix A for instructions.

- *Percent sag* on all products that gel. See Appendix A for instructions. All samples should be tested with the same cone and for the same length of time used to test the first sample.

Group 4 variations

Volume of the product is measured in millimeters using a graduated cylinder immediately after cooking is completed, and then the sample is used for subjective evaluation. Calculate the percent increase in volume as follows:

$$\% \text{ increase in volume} = \frac{\text{final volume}}{\text{initial volume}} \times 100$$

Subjective testing
Starches

Only visual testing is done in this experiment because the samples will become somewhat contaminated during the objective tests. In practice, the following characteristics should be evaluated:

Appearance (translucency, clarity, and color)
Rheological properties (flow of a sol or deformation characteristics of a gel, i.e., rigid, soft but not spreading).

Cereals and legumes

Appearance should focus on the distinctness of the outline of individual grains or pieces and also upon the color. Flavor comments should include unique flavor overtones and also the presence of any raw starch flavor. Mouthfeel descriptors might include harsh, mushy, distinct pieces, pleasing, pasty, or other terms that designate specific sensations in the mouth.

STUDY QUESTIONS

1. Describe the form in which starch is deposited in plants. Using this description, describe the process of gelatinization.

2. Is dextrinization a form of gelatinization? If not, explain the process of dextrinization.

3. Identify the optimum temperature for thickening each of the starches tested in the experiment.

4. Describe the process of gel formation, according to a presently accepted theory.

5. Why was the amount of flour used in the experiment greater than the amount of cornstarch used? Why was there a difference in the appearance of the flour-thickened paste and the cornstarch-thickened product?

Chart 2.1.1   Varying Concentrations of Various Starches

Starch	Highest temp. (°C)	Line spread Hot (mm)	Line spread Cold (mm)	Tenderness Penetrometer	% sag	Appearance
Waxy corn a. 16 g						
b. 8 g						
Corn c. 16 g						
d. 8 g						
Rice e. 16 g						
f. 8 g						
Quick tapioca g. 16 g						
h. 8 g						
Potato i. 16 g						
j. 8 g						
Wheat k. 16 g						
l. 8 g						
Ap flour m. 16 g						
n. 8 g						
Dextri. flour o. 16 g						

Name

ADDITIONAL OBSERVATIONS AND NOTES

CHART 2.1.2   TEMPERATURE OF MAXIMUM GELATINIZATION

Starch source	Line spread (mm)					Overall visual impression				
	70°C	80°C	90°C	95°C	Boiling	70°C	80°C	90°C	95°C	Boiling
a. Waxy corn										
b. Corn										
c. Rice										
d. Quick tapioca										
e. Potato										
f. Wheat										
g. AP flour										
h. Dextrin. flour										

ADDITIONAL OBSERVATIONS AND NOTES

CHART 2.1.3   EFFECT OF ACID AND SUGAR

Treatment	Line spread (mm)		Tenderness		Clarity	Rheological Characteristics
	Hot	Cold	Penetrometer	% sag		
Sugar a. 0 g*						
b. 25 g						
c. 50 g						
Lemon juice d. 30 ml, pH = _____						
e. 60 ml, pH = _____						
Sugar 25 g f. Lemon juice 30 ml						

*Control

Name

ADDITIONAL OBSERVATIONS AND NOTES

CHART 2.1.4   GELATINIZATION OF CEREALS AND LEGUMES

Treatment	Volume		Appearance	Flavor	Mouthfeel
	After cooking	% increase			
a. Minute rice					
b. Parboiled rice					
c. Polished rice (long grain)					
d. Polished rice (short grain)					
e. Instant oatmeal					
f. Quick oatmeal					
g. Regular oatmeal					
h. Navy beans					

Name

ADDITIONAL OBSERVATIONS AND NOTES

EXPERIMENT 2.2—STARCH-THICKENED PUDDINGS
OBJECTIVES

Upon completion of the experiment, you will be able to:

1. Describe the properties of modified and unmodified starches from corn when used in preparing a pudding.
2. Describe the properties of modified and unmodified waxy cornstarch when used in preparing a pudding.
3. Identify the factors to consider when selecting a starch for formulating a commercial pudding and explain the importance of each.
4. Select a specific starch well suited to preparing a milk-containing pudding and rationalize your choice.

BASIC FORMULA—PUDDING

24 g	Starch
65 g	Sugar
472 ml	Milk
5 ml	Vanilla
5 g	Butter

Thoroughly mix the starch and sugar in a 2-qt saucepan before gradually stirring in the milk to make a smooth slurry. Stir continuously while heating on medium high until mixture boils in the center of the pan. Add vanilla and butter, and stir to blend completely before pouring into 4 custard cups. Cover each with plastic wrap and chill 15 minutes in a pan of ice before testing.

1. **Type of starch**

   a. *Cornstarch (control)*—Prepare the basic formula, using cornstarch.

   b. *Waxy cornstarch*—Prepare the basic formula, using waxy cornstarch.

   c. *Cross-linked cornstarch*—Prepare the basic formula, using cross-linked cornstarch.

   d. *Cross-linked waxy cornstarch*—Prepare the basic formula, using cross-linked waxy cornstarch.

   e. *Rice starch*—Prepare the basic formula using rice starch.

   f. *Wheat starch*—Prepare the basic formula using wheat starch.

   g. *Quick tapioca*—Prepare the basic formula using quick tapioca.

   h. *Potato starch*—Prepare the basic formula using potato starch.

   i. *Arrowroot starch*—Prepare the basic formula using arrowroot starch.

    j. *Cornstarch and water*—Prepare the basic formula using cornstarch and using water instead of milk.

    k. *Waxy cornstarch and water*—Prepare the basic formula using waxy cornstarch and using water instead of milk.

    l. *Cross-linked cornstarch and water*—Prepare the basic formula using cross-linked cornstarch and using water instead of milk.

EVALUATION

Objective testing   Conduct penetrometer test on 1 cup if pudding gels. Perform a line spread test on pastes. Label and cover this sample tightly before placing in freezer for freeze-thaw stability observations after at least 24 hours of frozen storage. Freeze-thaw stability is judged by completely thawing samples, noting syneresis and textural properties.

Subjective testing   Evaluate the remaining cups of pudding, noting textural characteristics that can be observed visually and then checking flavor and mouthfeel. Note translucency of the samples made with water.

STUDY QUESTIONS

1. Which starches formed a gel? A sol? Do these results agree with what would be predicted from the literature? If not, how do you explain your results?

2. Compare the freeze-thaw stability of the various starches. Which starch exhibited the best freeze-thaw characteristics? Were there any other starches that were almost as satisfactory? If so, which were they?

3. Compare a root starch with a cereal starch when used for thickening.

4. Which of the cereal starches would you choose to use for thickening?

5. Compare the differences between cornstarch and waxy cornstarch for use as a thickening agent.

6. Compare the differences between cross-linked starches and their non-modified counterparts. Why does cross-linking influence starch properties?

CHART 2.2   STARCH-THICKENED PUDDINGS

Starch	Pene-trometer	Line spread	Appear-ance	Mouth-feel	Flavor	Freeze-thaw stability	
						Texture	Syneresis
a. Cornstarch (control)							
b. Waxy cornstarch							
c. Cross-linked cornstarch							
d. Cross-linked waxy cornstarch							
e. Rice							
f. Wheat							
g. Quick tapioca							
h. Potato							
i. Arrowroot							
j. Cornstarch + water							
k. Waxy cornstarch + water							
l. Cross-linked cornstarch + water							

Name

ADDITIONAL OBSERVATIONS AND NOTES

3
Fruits and Vegetables

Overall acceptability of cooked fruits and vegetables is influenced by possible changes in pigments, flavors, and texture. Cookery methods for various fruits and vegetables can be selected to provide optimal palatability while also maintaining useful levels of nutrients.

The pigments in fruits and vegetables are classified in three major categories:

- Chlorophyll
- Carotenoids
- Flavonoids

Within each of these three large categories are subdivisions. The most striking of the subdivisions is found in the flavonoids, the category that includes a large group of the white to yellow-pigmented anthoxanthins and the group of purple to blue compounds classified as anthocyanins. The pH of the cooking medium can cause changes in the color of the chlorophyll and flavonoid pigments. Time is also a factor in determining the color of vegetables containing chlorophyll. Experiments with the pH and the cooking time of vegetables serve to illustrate these changes.

Flavor is an important characteristic in determining the acceptability of fruits and vegetables. Cookery methods can be selected to minimize or to optimize flavors. The length of time a vegetable is cooked and the amount of water used will influence flavor in the finished vegetable. Other factors are the retention of volatile compounds and the cooking temperatures.

The texture of a fruit or vegetable can enhance the acceptability of the food when the factors influencing softening are controlled. These factors include:

- pH of the cooking medium
- Control of osmotic pressure
- Control of salts in the cooking medium
- Length of cooking time

EXPERIMENT 3.1—PIGMENTS
OBJECTIVES

Upon completion of the experiment, you will be able to:

1. Identify the pigment categories and the color of each in acidic and alkaline media.
2. Explain the conversion of chlorophyll pigments to pheophytins as a function of time and pH.
3. Discuss the effect of various cooking methods, such as use of a lid, a pressure cooker, and microwave oven on vegetable pigments.
4. Determine the effect of the use of a lid and of various types of water on the pH of the cooking medium.

SAMPLE PREPARATION

1. **Vegetable and fruit pigments at various pH levels**

    a. *Chlorophyll*—Pour 10 ml of a buffered solution of pH 3 into a test tube. Repeat with 10 ml of buffered solutions into 3 other test tubes: pH 5, pH 7, and pH 8. Weigh out 13 g of dried spinach. After grinding it thoroughly with a mortar and pestle, add 52 ml of acetone and 13 ml water. Grind again with the mortar and pestle before filtering. With an eyedropper, drop the filtrate into the test tube containing the pH 3 solution. Count the number of drops required to change the color of the solution. Put this same number of drops of filtrate into each of the other 3 test tubes. Pour a small amount of each solution into clean test tubes labeled with the designated pH (3, 5, 7, and 8) and place these on display. Place the original 4 test tubes in a boiling water bath for 10 minutes.

    b. *Carotenoids*—Grate 95 g of carrots (pared). Place in a blender with 95 ml of water and whirl for 2 minutes. Filter the slurry. Arrange the test tubes in the same manner as for procedure 1a above. Add the filtrate with an eyedropper, counting the drops added until the color changes in the pH 3 tube. Put the same number of drops into the pH 5, pH 7, and pH 8 tubes. Pour a small amount of each of these samples into appropriately labeled, clean test tubes and place them on display. Place the 4 original tubes in a boiling water bath for 10 minutes.

    c. *Anthocyanin*—Grate 95 g red cabbage (or chop it fine). Place in a blender with 95 ml water, and whirl for 2 minutes. Filter the slurry. Arrange the test tubes in the same manner as in procedure 1a. Add the filtrate as in 1a, but add to pH 8 tube until the color changes. Pour a small amount of each solution into clean test tubes labeled with the designated pH (3, 5, 7, 8) and place these on display. Place the original 4 test tubes in a boiling water bath for 10 minutes.

BASIC FORMULA—BROCCOLI

2 lb Broccoli

Wash the broccoli well. Chop all of the stalks and flowers into segments about 1/2″ long and approximately 1/3″ diameter. Place the entire mixture in a large mixing bowl and stir to blend the stalks and flowers uniformly throughout.

Randomly remove 50 g of the chopped broccoli for each of the following preparations. Cook the broccoli according to the variation assigned. After cooking, remove the broccoli from the cooking liquid with a slotted spoon. Pour the cooking liquid into a glass beaker and place beside the plate of broccoli for evaluation. When the cooking liquid has cooled to room temperature, test the pH on the pH meter. If pH paper is being used, the test may be made before the liquid cools.

2. **Varying cooking methods**

a. *Lid on, 5 minutes*—In a covered 1-qt saucepan bring 250 ml of water to a boil; add chopped broccoli. Boil 5 minutes.

b. *Lid on, 15 minutes*—In a covered 1-qt saucepan bring 250 ml of water to a boil; add 50 g chopped broccoli. Boil 15 minutes.

c. *Lid off, 5 minutes*—In an uncovered 1-qt saucepan bring 250 ml water to a boil. Add 50 g chopped broccoli. Boil 5 minutes.

d. *Lid off, 15 minutes*—In an uncovered 1-qt saucepan bring 250 ml water to a boil. Add 50 g chopped broccoli. Boil 15 minutes.

e. *Cold water start, lid off*—In an uncovered 1-qt saucepan, place 250 ml cold tap water and 50 g of broccoli. Heat (uncovered) to a boil and continue to boil actively for 5 minutes. Note total time for heating and boiling.

f. *Distilled water, lid off*—In an uncovered 1-qt saucepan, heat 250 ml distilled water to a boil; add 50 g chopped broccoli. Boil 5 minutes.

g. *Pressure saucepan, 2 minutes*—Place 250 ml tap water and 50 g broccoli in a pressure saucepan. Follow the directions for the pressure saucepan to achieve 15 pounds of pressure. Maintain pressure for 2 minutes. **Warning:** Cool according to directions before opening pressure saucepan.

h. *Pressure saucepan, 10 minutes*—Repeat 2g, but maintain 15 pounds pressure for 10 minutes before cooling the pressure saucepan according to directions.

i. *Microwave oven, uncovered*—Place 50 g chopped broccoli in a small dish. Add 15 ml water. Cook in microwave oven for 1 minute and 30 seconds.

j. *Microwave oven, covered*—Repeat 2i, but cook in a small, covered casserole dish.

k. *Steamer*—Place 50 g chopped broccoli in a covered steamer containing enough water to boil throughout the steaming period, but without touching the broccoli. Note the time required for the stalks to become fork tender.

EVALUATION

1. Note the colors of the buffered solutions for each of the pigments at each pH being tested; notations should be made before and after heating the pigments.

2. Record the pH of the cooking liquid from each of the broccoli variations being tested. Note the color of the cooking liquid and also the color of the vegetable.

STUDY QUESTIONS

1. Name the 3 pigment categories and the major subdivisions of the flavonoids; identify the color of the pigments in acid and alkaline pH ranges.

2. Do any of the pigments change color when heated for an extended period of time? If so, which? Explain the reaction.

3. Compare the pH of the various cooking liquids from the broccoli variations.

   a. Does boiling modify the pH? If so, how?

   b. Is there any difference in the pH of the distilled water and tap water? If so, what is the difference?

   c. Does the pH of the cooking liquid change when a vegetable is heated in it? If so, what causes the change?

   d. Does use of a lid influence the pH of the cooking liquid? If so, why?

   e. Is the color of broccoli the same when cooked in a pressure cooker at 15 pounds pressure for 2 minutes as it is at 10 minutes?

   f. Does microwave cookery influence the color of chlorophyll? Give an explanation for your answer.

   g. Does covering the vegetable in microwave cookery modify chlorophyll color? Explain your answer.

CHART 3.1.1   PIGMENTS—EXTRACTION REACTIONS

Pigment	Color before heating solution				Color after heating solution (10 minutes)			
	pH 3	pH 5	pH 7	pH 8	pH 3	pH 5	pH 7	pH 8
1a. Chlorophyll								
1b. Carotinoid								
Flavonoids 1c. Anthocyanin								
1d. Anthoxanthin								

ADDITIONAL OBSERVATIONS AND NOTES

CHART 3.1.2   EFFECT OF COOKERY METHODS ON CHLOROPHYLL

Treatment	Cooking liquid		Vegetable color
	pH	Color	
a. Lid on, 5 min.			
b. Lid on, 15 min.			
c. Lid off, 5 min.			
d. Lid off, 15 min.			
e. Cold water start, lid off, time: _____			
f. Distilled water, lid off			
g. Pressure saucepan, 2 min.			
h. Pressure saucepan, 10 min.			
i. Microwave, uncovered			
j. Microwave, covered			
k. Steamer			

Name

ADDITIONAL OBSERVATIONS AND NOTES

EXPERIMENT 3.2—FLAVOR OF VEGETABLES
OBJECTIVES

Upon completion of the experiment, you will be able to:

1. Explain the effect of various cooking treatments on the flavor of mild-flavored vegetables.
2. Explain the effect of various cooking treatments on the flavor of strong-flavored vegetables.
3. Discuss the interrelationship of volatile flavoring compounds and cooking methods.

PROCEDURE

1. **Carrots (mild-flavored vegetable)**—Wash and pare carrots. Cut into matchstick pieces about 2″ long × 1/2″ across. For each of the methods outlined below, weigh 100 g of sliced carrots. Prepare according to assigned directions and serve for subjective evaluation of flavor. Note boiling times carefully.

   a. *Waterless, covered*—Place 100 g of carrots and 25 ml water in a very heavy saucepan with a tightly fitting lid. Heat to boiling and continue boiling just until fork tender. Watch carefully and add water as necessary to prevent scorching. Note the time required.

   b. *100 ml water, covered*—Place 100 ml water in a 1-qt saucepan. Heat quickly to boiling before adding carrots. Immediately add 100 g of carrots and boil gently until fork tender. Note the boiling time required.

   c. *300 ml water, covered*—Prepare as in 1b, except use 300 ml water. Note the boiling time required.

   d. *100 ml water, uncovered*—Prepare as in 1b, except cook without a cover. Note the boiling time required.

   e. *300 ml water, uncovered*—Heat 300 ml water to boiling. Add 100 g carrots and boil without a cover until tender. Note time required.

   f. *Tender + 10 minutes, covered*—Prepare as in 1c, but continue to boil 10 minutes after the carrots are fork tender. Note total time.

   g. *Cold start, uncovered*—Place 150 ml water and 100 g carrots in an uncovered 1-qt saucepan. Bring to a boil and continue boiling until tender. Note total cooking time.

   h. *Stir-fry*—Briefly heat 5 ml salad oil in a wok or heavy frying pan and add 100 g carrots. Stir briefly; cover the wok lifting the cover to stir every 30 seconds. If carrots start to burn, add 10 ml water. Cook just until tender. Note the cooking time.

   i. *Microwave oven*—Place 100 g carrots and 25 ml water in a small, covered casserole dish. Place in microwave oven and cook for 1 minute and 30 seconds. Stir the carrots and cook covered another minute and 30 seconds.

    j. *Pressure saucepan*—Place 100 g carrots and 150 ml water in pressure saucepan. Heat the saucepan to 15 pounds pressure and maintain pressure for 1 1/2 minutes. Cool pressure saucepan quickly under cold running water to reduce the pressure and avoid overcooking. **Warning:** Do not open pressure saucepan until cooled sufficiently to relieve the pressure.

    k. *Steamer*—Place 100 g carrots in steamer and add enough water to boil throughout the cooking period without being high enough to touch the carrots. Note the time required.

2. **Onions (strong-flavored vegetable)**—Wash and peel onions, trimming off both ends and then cutting into wedges. Prepare methods a through k (above), using 100 g of onion. Prepare according to directions and serve for subjective evaluation of flavor.

3. **Cabbage (strong-flavored vegetable)**—Wash cabbage thoroughly and remove any damaged outer leaves. Cut into very thin wedges. Prepare methods a through k (above), using 100 g of cabbage. Prepare according to directions and serve for subjective evaluation of flavor.

4. **Potatoes (starch-containing vegetable)**—Cut potatoes into 1″ cubes. Prepare methods a through k (above) using 100 g of potatoes. Prepare according to directions and serve for subjective evaluation of flavor.

EVALUATION

Evaluate each treatment of each vegetable, noting particularly the intensity of odor and flavor for each treatment. When possible, identify descriptive words to help characterize the qualities noted. Ignore textural differences and color. Concentrate on odor and flavor only.

STUDY QUESTIONS

1. What is the effect on flavor when mild-flavored vegetables are boiled in a limited amount of water?

2. What is the effect on flavor when strong-flavored vegetables are boiled in a limited amount of water?

3. What is the effect of prolonged cooking time on the flavor of onions as compared with cabbage?

4. Compare the odor and flavor characteristics of vegetables cooked in the pressure saucepan, the wok, the microwave oven, and the steamer. Which method produces the mildest flavor? Which produces the flavor that is most pleasing and typical of the vegetable?

5. Does the cooking method have a strong influence on the flavor of vegetables containing relatively high levels of starch? What guidelines might be suggested to promote optimum flavor in cooked vegetables containing relatively high levels of starch?

CHART 3.2.1   ODOR AND FLAVOR OF CARROTS AND ONIONS

Treatment	Carrots			Onions		
	Time	Odor	Flavor	Time	Odor	Flavor
a. Waterless, covered						
b. 100 ml water, covered						
c. 300 ml water, covered						
d. 100 ml water, uncovered						
e. 300 ml water, uncovered						
f. Tender + 10 min., covered						
g. Cold start, uncovered						
h. Stir-fry						
i. Microwave oven						
j. Pressure saucepan						
k. Steamer						

Name

ADDITIONAL OBSERVATIONS AND NOTES

CHART 3.2.2 ODOR AND FLAVOR OF CABBAGE AND POTATOES

Treatment	Cabbage			Potatoes		
	Time	Odor	Flavor	Time	Odor	Flavor
a. Waterless, covered						
b. 100 ml water, covered						
c. 300 ml water, covered						
d. 100 ml water, uncovered						
e. 300 ml water, uncovered						
f. Tender + 10 min., covered						
g. Cold start, uncovered						
h. Stir-fry						
i. Microwave oven						
j. Pressure saucepan						
k. Steamer						

Name

ADDITIONAL OBSERVATIONS AND NOTES

EXPERIMENT 3.3—TEXTURE OF VEGETABLES AND FRUITS
OBJECTIVES

Upon completion of the experiment, you will be able to:

1. Predict the effect of the use of acid and alkali in the softening of vegetable and fruit tissues and interpret the appropriate theory.
2. Interpret the role of calcium salts in determining the texture of cooked plant products.
3. Define osmotic pressure and illustrate how it may be used to advantage in the storage of vegetables and the cooking of fruits.

PROCEDURE

1. **Cooking media and texture**—Wash cauliflower thoroughly and break into flowerets. Prepare each of the following using 80 g cauliflower for each treatment. Note the pH of the cooking medium. Drain well and serve for evaluation of texture.

    a. *Soda, 3 minutes*—In a covered 1-qt saucepan, heat 350 ml of water to a boil. Add 0.5 g baking soda and 80 g of cauliflower. Quickly return to boiling and boil 3 minutes. Drain and serve for evaluation.

    b. *Soda, 20 minutes*—Repeat 1a, but boil for 20 minutes.

    c. *Vinegar, 3 minutes*—In a covered 1-qt saucepan, bring 350 ml water to a boil. Add 30 ml vinegar and 80 g cauliflower. Quickly return to a boil and boil 3 minutes. Drain and serve for evaluation.

    d. *Vinegar, 20 minutes*—Repeat 1c, but boil 20 minutes.

    e. *Lemon juice, 3 minutes*—Repeat 1c, but replace vinegar with 30 ml lemon juice and boil 3 minutes.

    f. *Lemon juice, 20 minutes*—Repeat 1c, but replace vinegar with 30 ml lemon juice and boil 20 minutes.

    g. *Cream of tartar, 3 minutes*—Repeat 1c, but replace the vinegar with 1.0 g cream of tartar and boil 3 minutes.

    h. *Cream of tartar, 20 minutes*—Repeat 1c, but replace the vinegar with 1.0 g cream of tartar and boil 20 minutes.

    i. *Tap water, 3 minutes (control)*—Repeat 1a, but do not add soda. Boil 3 minutes.

    j. *Milk, 20 minutes*—Repeat 1a, but using milk in place of water; boil 20 minutes, being careful to avoid boiling over.

2. **Softening of legumes**—Wash navy beans. Weigh out 50 g dry beans for each treatment. Prepare according to the outlined procedures; carefully drain the legumes from the cooking liquid. Check the pH of the cooking liquid. Note cooking time to tenderize beans.

a. *Overnight soak*—Place 50 g dried navy beans in 475 ml water; let stand overnight. Drain and weigh the soaked beans. Add 236 ml fresh water. Simmer in covered saucepan until tender. Note the cooking time required for the beans to become tender. Drain and serve for evaluation. Note the pH of the cooking liquid.

b. *Overnight soak, 0.5 g soda*—Soak and prepare as described in 2a, except add 0.5 g baking soda to the water used for soaking overnight. (The soda water is removed and discarded when the beans are drained prior to weighing.) Cook beans in 236 ml fresh water until tender. Drain and serve for evaluation. Note the pH of the cooking liquid.

c. *Overnight soak, 45 ml vinegar*—Prepare as described in 1a, except add 45 ml vinegar to the soaking water. (The vinegar is removed when the beans are drained prior to weighing.) Cook in 236 ml fresh water until tender. Drain and serve for evaluation. Measure the pH of the cooking liquid.

d. *Overnight soak, distilled water*—Prepare as in 2a, except use distilled water rather than tap water both for the soaking and cooking water.

e. *No soak*—Place 50 g dried navy beans in 475 ml water. Simmer in a covered saucepan until the beans are tender. Note the cooking time required. Drain and serve for evaluation. Note the pH of the cooking liquid.

f. *No soak, 0.5 g soda*—Prepare as described in 2e, but add 0.5 g soda to the cooking water.

g. *No soak, 45 ml vinegar*—Prepare as described in 2e, but add 45 ml vinegar to the cooking water.

h. *Overnight soak, 45 ml molasses*—Prepare as described in 2e, but add 45 ml molasses to the cooking water.

i. *Soak overnight, pressure saucepan*—Soak beans overnight, as described in 2a. Drain off water and weigh beans. Place beans and 236 ml water in a pressure saucepan. Following manufacturer's directions, heat to 15 pounds pressure and maintain pressure for 35 minutes cooking time. Cool under cold, running water to reduce pressure before opening the pressure saucepan. If beans are not tender, estimate approximately how much more time will be needed, and continue to cook at 15 lb pressure until done. Note the cooking time and the pH of the cooking liquid.

j. *No soak, pressure saucepan*—Place 475 ml water and 50 g dried beans in a pressure saucepan. Following manufacturer's directions, heat to 15 lb pressure and maintain that pressure for 40 minutes. Cool as described in 2i. Continue cooking, if not done. Note cooking time and pH of cooking liquid.

k. *Soak overnight, slow cooker*—Place 50 g of beans and 475 ml water over night, as described in 2a. Drain off the water and weigh the beans. Place beans in a slow cooker. Cook on low setting for 10 hours. If necessary, continue cooking until tender, noting time required. If preferred, use the high setting for at least 4 hours or until tender. Note total cooking time and the pH of the cooking liquid.

   l. *No soak, slow cooker*—Place 50 g of beans and 475 ml water in a slow cooker. Cook on low setting for 10 hours. If preferred, use the high setting for at least 5 hours or until tender. Note total cooking time and the pH of the cooking liquid.

3. **Storage of succulents**—Wash lettuce thoroughly. Store 2 leaves in each of the following ways for at least 8 hours. Remove from storage for evaluation.

   a. *Uncovered, room temperature*—Place lettuce leaves on counter (uncovered) at room temperature for at least 8 hours.

   b. *Uncovered, large refrigerator compartment*—Place lettuce leaves (uncovered) in the main section of the refrigerator, and store for at least 8 hours.

   c. *Hydrator drawer*—Place lettuce leaves (unwrapped) in the hydrator drawer, being careful to close the drawer tightly. Store at least 8 hours.

   d. *Salt water*—Place lettuce leaves in a bowl containing 236 ml water and 1 g salt. Store at least 8 hours in the refrigerator.

   e. *Ice water*—Place lettuce leaves in a bowl containing 236 ml water and 5 ice cubes. Be sure lettuce is immersed. Cover with aluminum foil. Store in refrigerator in the bowl for at least 8 hours.

4. **Use of osmotic pressure**—Wash and pare apples before coring and slicing into rings.

   a. *Water only (control)*—Place 236 ml water in a 1-qt saucepan and heat to boiling. Add 1/3 of the apple slices; simmer just until tender. Note the cooking time.

   b. *Dilute sugar syrup*—In a 1-qt saucepan, simmer 100 g sugar and 236 ml water with 1/3 of the apple slices. Simmer until apples are tender and translucent. Note the cooking time required.

   c. *Concentrated sugar syrup*—In a 1-qt saucepan, simmer 300 g sugar and 236 ml water with the apple slices. Simmer until apples are tender. Note the cooking time.

EVALUATION

1. Note the pH of the cooking liquid remaining from each of the treatments in Procedure 1. Note the relationship between cooking time and pH of the cooking medium in influencing the tenderizing of vegetable structure. Evaluate texture from the standpoint of acceptability. Note the influence of salt on texture.

2. Note the times required to achieve tender beans and the methods that resulted in the differences. Beans should be tender, but not mushy. Note also the pH of the cooking liquids.

3. Observe the relative crispness of the lettuce leaves stored under different conditions. Crispness can be evaluated easily by folding over part of the leaf and listening to the sound. The sense of feel also helps to detect crispness.

4. Note the translucency of the apples, their plumpness, and their ability to hold their shape. Tenderness and flavor are other attributes to judge. After tasting each sample, exhale vigorously and see whether the flavor or aftertaste shows any variation as a result. This test is for detecting aftertaste.

STUDY QUESTIONS

1. Why does the pH of the cooking medium influence the texture of cooked fruits and vegetables? What cookery methods should be employed to ensure adequate, but not excessive, softening of cells?

2. Are vinegar, lemon juice, and cream of tartar advantageous in vegetable cookery? Is soda? Explain your answers.

3. Does milk influence softening of vegetable tissues? Why?

4. Is it absolutely essential to soak navy beans before cooking them?

5. What techniques can be employed to soften navy beans more quickly while still achieving a desirable finished product? What precautions might need to be taken in using any of these techniques?

6. What are the differences between using a slow cooker and a pressure saucepan for cooking dried navy beans?

7. Why is cold storage in a moist environment advantageous in achieving crispness in succulents? Why is salt water detrimental? Would sugar be predicted to have an effect similar to salt when added to water used for storing succulents? Explain your answer.

8. When is storage of succulents in ice water appropriate? Is this the way usually preferred when lettuce is to be stored for several days? If not, what storage method is recommended?

9. What is the effect of cooking apple rings in water? Why does this happen?

10. What is the effect of cooking apple rings in a dilute sugar syrup? In a concentrated sugar syrup? Explain why each occurs.

CHART 3.3.1   COOKING MEDIA AND TEXTURE OF CAULIFLOWER

Treatment	pH of medium	Color	Texture
Soda (0.5 g) a. 3 min.			
b. 20 min.			
Vinegar (30 ml) c. 3 min.			
d. 20 min.			
Lemon juice (30 ml) e. 3 min.			
f. 20 min.			
Cream of tartar (1 g) g. 3 min.			
h. 20 min.			
Tap water* i. 3 min.			
Milk j. 20 min.			

*Control

Name

ADDITIONAL OBSERVATIONS AND NOTES

CHART 3.3.2 SOFTENING OF LEGUMES (NAVY BEANS)

Treatment	Weight soaked beans (g)	Cooking time (hr. min.)	pH of cooking liquid	Texture
Overnight soak a. No additive				
b. 0.5 g soda				
c. 45 ml vinegar				
d. distilled water				
No soak e. No additive	XXX			
f. 0.5 g soda	XXX			
g. 45 ml vinegar	XXX			
Soak h. 45 ml molasses	XXX			
Pressure saucepan i. Soak overnight				
j. No soak	XXX			
Slow cooker k. Soak overnight				
l. No soak	XXX			

ADDITIONAL OBSERVATIONS AND NOTES

CHART 3.3.3   STORAGE OF SUCCULENTS (LETTUCE)

Treatment	Crispness of texture evaluated by:	
	Sound	**Feel**
a. Uncovered, room temp. storage		
b. Uncovered, stored in large compartment of refrigerator		
c. Hydrator drawer, refrigerator*		
d. Salt water, covered, refrigerator		
e. Ice water, refrigerator		

*Control

Name

ADDITIONAL OBSERVATIONS AND NOTES

CHART 3.3.4   OSMOTIC PRESSURE AND TEXTURE OF APPLES

Treatment	Cooking time (min.)	Appearance	Texture	Flavor and aftertaste
a. Water only*				
b. Dilute sugar syrup (1 part sugar to 2 parts water)				
c. Concentrated sugar syrup (1 1/2 parts sugar to 1 part water)				

*Control

ADDITIONAL OBSERVATIONS AND NOTES

4
Fats and Oils

Technology in fats and oils has been developing at a very rapid rate, partly as a response to the needs of the food industry and partly to meet consumer demands for products geared to satisfy nutritional concerns. The diversity of products now available to consumers makes it particularly important that experiments be included in this manual to demonstrate the performance qualities that can be expected from various choices.

Fats are utilized for a range of products in the consumer market. Uses include spreads for bread and bread products, cooking medium in shallow and deep fat frying, ingredient in emulsions such as salad dressings, and as a shortening or tenderizing ingredient in a range of baked products. The performance expectations in these various capacities are quite different, and no single product is capable of providing maximum quality in all of these roles.

The experiments in this chapter are designed to demonstrate (1) the compositional differences, (2) the range in melting point and plasticity, (3) the smoke point and fat absorption involved in deep fat frying, and (4) the contributions of fats and oils in emulsion formation and (5) the tenderizing of baked products. The experiments will also draw attention to the importance of fats and oils in influencing the flavor of products.

To gain a broader understanding of the value of the various products, students are encouraged to relate performance characteristics seen in the experiments to the nutritional merits of the various fats and oils. Cost factors also need to be recognized to round out the picture regarding appropriate choices of fats and oils in creating and/or preparing various foods.

EXPERIMENT 4.1—MELTING POINTS AND COMPOSITION
OBJECTIVES

Upon completion of the experiment, you will be able to:

1. Identify differences in content of the various fat products in the market.
2. Differentiate between the use of diet margarines, whipped margarines, soft, and regular margarines.
3. Evaluate the plastic range of the various fats tested.
4. Select the best fat product for specific uses.

PROCEDURE

1. **Record**—Record the label information for each fat being tested (Chart 4.1.1).

2. **Melting point and fat content**—Lightly pack the assigned margarine into a 1/4-cup metal measure, and level it carefully with the straight edge of a spatula. Place the measuring cup in a frying pan. Position the frying pan on a heating unit on the range, but do not turn on the unit. Position a ring stand supporting a thermometer so that the bulb of the thermometer will be in the center of the fat. The bulb must be covered completely by the fat, but not touching the bottom of the cup. This positioning needs to be done carefully. Without splattering on the fat, carefully pour cold water into the frying pan to a depth of 1/4".

   Begin heating very slowly. Note the temperature when fat at the edge of the cup melts. Continue heating very slowly until all of the fat is melted. At precisely the point where all the fat melts, note the temperature. Very carefully remove the cup from the frying pan, and pour the melted fat into a graduated cylinder. If it is necessary to use a funnel to do this, be sure the funnel is warm enough to keep the fat from solidifying. Note the volume of the melted fat. After the measurement is taken, insert the thermometer and observe changes in the fat as it cools.

   Note any layering that may appear and the volume of the layers. At precisely the point that the fat loses its ability to flow when the cylinder is tipped, record the temperature and remove the thermometer. Allow the fat to continue cooling without disturbance. Observe the appearance of the modified fat. To remove the fat, place the cylinder in hot water until the fat melts enough around the edges to slide out.

   a. *Butter*—Using butter, follow the directions above.

   b. *Regular corn oil margarine*—Using regular corn oil margarine, follow the directions above.

   c. *Regular canola oil margarine*—Using regular canola oil margarine, follow the directions above.

   d. *Regular safflower oil margarine*—Using regular safflower oil margarine, follow the directions above.

e. *Regular soybean oil margarine*—Using regular soybean oil margarine, follow the directions above.

f. *Benecol®*—Using Benecol®, follow the directions above.

g. *Take Control®*—Using Take Control®, follow the directions above.

h. *Soft margarine (corn oil)*—Using soft corn oil margarine, follow the directions above.

i. *Soft margarine (safflower or other oil)*—Using soft margarine (safflower or other oil), follow the directions above.

j. *Diet margarine*—Using diet margarine, follow the directions above.

k. *Diet margarine no. 2*—Using a different diet margarine, follow the directions above.

l. *Whipped butter*—Using whipped butter, follow the directions above.

m. *Lard*—Using lard, follow the directions above.

n. *Shortening*—Using shortening, follow the directions above.

o. *Additional products*—If additional products are being tested, follow the directions above.

3. **Plasticity**—Pack a 1/4-cup measuring cup with the assigned fat. Level with a spatula. Allow the measured fat to sit at room temperature for 30 minutes. Using the needle attachment on the penetrometer, test the penetration by releasing the needle for precisely 2 seconds. Transfer the margarine to the refrigerator for 30 minutes. Test again on the penetrometer. Place the fat in the freezer for 30 minutes; again take the penetrometer reading. Be sure to check the temperature of the fat immediately following each penetrometer test. Smooth the surface of the fat with a spatula after the thermometer has been removed. Save the fat for Experiment 4.2.

EVALUATION

1. Compare not only the initial temperature at which melting begins and the final temperature, but also the total temperature span over which melting occurs for the various fats. Review these data carefully for commonalities within the specific groups of fats and for other generalizations that may be drawn from the results. Compare total volume of regular butter with its whipped counterpart. Observe the amount of water found in the various fats as they cool and separate. Look carefully at the crystalline nature of each of the re-solidified fats.

2. Compare the penetrometer results with the trends in melting points observed.

STUDY QUESTIONS

1. Which fats used in this experiment contained the largest amount of water? The least?

2. What are the possible reasons for incorporating water into a fat? How does the water content influence the ways in which a fat can be used in food preparation?

3. Does butter have as wide a range between initial and final melting temperature as does a regular margarine? How does this difference influence the usefulness of butter? Of margarine?

4. Do Benecol® and Take Control® exhibit the same characteristics as butter? As margarine?

5. What is done commercially to avoid the coarse crystal structure observed in the fats that were heated and then cooled in this experiment? Why is it important to have smaller crystals in fats?

6. Which fats were softest at room temperature? At refrigerator temperature? At freezer temperature? How can this information be applied in food preparation?

7. Does the order of the ingredients on the label provide clues as to probable physical characteristics of fats? Explain your answer.

CHART 4.1.1 LABEL INFORMATION ON FATS

Fat (type)	Brand name	Cost/lb.	Calories/tbsp.	Ingredients (in order listed on label)
a. Butter				
b. Reg. margarine (corn oil)				
c. Reg. margarine (canola oil)				
d. Reg. margarine (safflower)				
e. Reg. margarine (soybean)				
f. Benecol®				
g. Take Control®				
h. Soft margarine (corn oil)				
i. Soft margarine (oil)				
j. Diet margarine (oil)				
k. Diet margarine (oil)				
l. Whipped butter				
m. Lard				
n. Shortening ( )				
o. Other ( )				

Name

ADDITIONAL OBSERVATIONS AND NOTES

CHART 4.1.2   MELTING POINT AND FAT CONTENT

Fat	Melting point			Volume		Temp. of solidification (°C)	Appearance of solidified fat
	Initial (°C)	Final (°C)	Range (°C)	Total (ml)	Water (ml)		
a. Butter							
b. Reg. margarine (corn oil)							
c. Reg. margarine (canola oil)							
d. Reg. margarine (safflower)							
e. Reg. margarine (soybean)							
f. Benecol®							
g. Take Control®							
h. Soft margarine (corn oil)							
i. Soft margarine (oil)							
j. Diet margarine (oil)							
k. Diet margarine (oil)							
l. Whipped butter							
m. Lard							
n. Shortening ( )							
o. Other ( )							

Name

ADDITIONAL OBSERVATIONS AND NOTES

CHART 4.1.3   PLASTICITY AS INDICATED BY PENETROMETER READINGS

Fat	Room temp.		Refrig. temp.		Freezer temp.	
	Pene. (mm)	Fat temp. (°C)	Pene. (mm)	Fat temp. (°C)	Pene. (mm)	Fat temp. (°C)
a. Butter						
b. Reg. margarine (corn oil)						
c. Reg. margarine (canola oil)						
d. Reg. margarine (safflower)						
e. Reg. margarine (soybean)						
f. Benecol®						
g. Take Control®						
h. Soft margarine (corn oil)						
i. Soft margarine (oil)						
j. Diet margarine (oil)						
k. Diet margarine (oil)						
l. Whipped butter						
m. Lard						
n. Shortening ( )						
o. Other ( )						

Name

ADDITIONAL OBSERVATIONS AND NOTES

EXPERIMENT 4.2—FRYING, ABSORPTION, AND SMOKE POINT OBJECTIVES

Upon completion of the experiment, you will be able to:

1. Identify factors that influence the smoke points of fats.
2. Discuss the significance of temperature of the fat in influencing fat absorption during deep fat frying.
3. Outline the factors to be considered in selecting a fat for use in deep fat frying.
4. Review the reasons for selecting a specific temperature or for avoiding other temperatures in deep fat frying.
5. Identify the changes that take place in a fat over a period of time when it is used for deep fat frying.

PROCEDURE

1. **Smoke points**—Place 1/4 c of the assigned fat in a clean, dry metal can from which the label has been removed. Securely position the can on a gas or electric burner so that it cannot tip. Use a ring stand to hold a laboratory thermometer with the bulb immersed in the fat, but not touching the bottom of the can. Begin heating the fat when everything is positioned securely and a portable fire extinguisher is handy. Heat the fat until the fat begins to smoke. Smoke can be observed most easily by holding a dark piece of paper at a distance away from the burner so that it serves as a background, but is not a potential fire hazard. As soon as the smoke is rising, note the temperature. Turn off the heat and let the fat cool without moving it.

   a. *Butter*—Remove water from the butter by warming the butter in a small pan until it melts and the fat separates from the water and milk solids. (Water is removed to avoid splattering when the butter is heated to high temperatures in the experiment.) Transfer the yellow butter to the can and follow procedure 1 described in the preceding paragraph.

   b. *Regular corn oil margarine*—Using regular corn oil margarine, follow the directions in 1a (butter), including removing the water.

   c. *Soft margarine (corn oil)*—Using soft margarine (corn oil), follow the directions for 1a (butter), including removing the water.

   d. *Diet margarine*—Using diet margarine, follow the directions for 1a (butter), including removing the water.

   e. *Benecol®*—Using Benecol®, follow the directions for 1a (butter), including removing the water.

   f. *Take Control®*—Using Take Control®, follow the directions for 1a (butter), including removing the water.

g. *Lard*—Using lard, follow procedure 1. (Omit step for removing water.)

h. *Shortening*—Using shortening, follow procedure 1. (Omit step for removing water.)

i. *Corn oil*—Using corn oil, follow procedure 1.

j. *Safflower oil*—Using safflower oil, follow procedure 1.

k. *Peanut oil*—Using peanut oil, follow procedure 1.

2. **Fat absorption during deep fat frying**—Using the type of oil assigned, determine the length of time required for 50 ml of the oil to drain from a burette. (This is not done with the shortening variation.) With a doughnut cutter, cut a "doughnut" from each slice of bread. In a 1-qt saucepan, place 454 g fat or 472 ml of the oil assigned. Use a ring stand to position a deep fat frying or laboratory thermometer so that the bulb is immersed in the fat or oil, but not touching the bottom of the pan. Begin to heat the fat. While the fat is being heated, weigh one of the doughnuts and record its weight.

When the temperature of the fat reaches 163°C (325°F), transfer the weighed doughnut into the hot fat with a spatula, being careful not to splash the fat. Begin timing immediately. Care must be taken to maintain the frying temperature of 163°C. As soon as the doughnut is a pleasing brown on the bottom, use a chopstick to turn to brown the other side. When the second side is a pleasing brown, remove the doughnut, using the chopstick to remove and suspend the doughnut over the hot fat to allow excess fat to drip into the pan. Note the total time required to fry the doughnut. Weigh the doughnut; calculate the difference between the initial and the fried weight.

While heating the fat to the next frying temperature of 177°C (350°F), weigh the next doughnut to be fried. Follow the frying procedures outlined above. Repeat the process for the doughnut to be fried at 190°C (375°F) and for the doughnut to be fried at 204°C (400°F).

Let the fat cool before measuring flow time for 50 ml oil through the burette.

a. *Corn oil*—Using the basic procedure outlined above, fry 4 doughnuts in corn oil.

b. *Peanut oil*—Using the basic procedure outlined above, fry 4 doughnuts in peanut oil.

c. *Shortening*—Using the basic procedure outlined above, fry 4 doughnuts in shortening.

d. *Old oil used at least 3 hours for frying*—Using the basic procedure outlined above, fry 4 doughnuts in oil that has been used previously for at least 3 hours for frying.

e. *Old oil and fresh oil*—Using the basic procedure outlined above, fry 4 doughnuts in a half and half mixture of oil that has been used at least 3 hours for frying and fresh oil (corn or peanut).

CHART 4.2.1   SMOKE POINTS

Treatment	Smoke Point (°C)	Observations
a. Butter		
b. Regular corn oil margarine		
c. Soft corn oil margarine		
d. Diet margarine		
e. Benecol®		
f. Take Control®		
g. Lard		
h. Shortening		
i. Corn oil		
j. Safflower oil		
k. Peanut oil		

Name

ADDITIONAL OBSERVATIONS AND NOTES

CHART 4.2.2 FAT ABSORPTION AND DEEP FAT FRYING OF DOUGHNUTS

Treatment	Weight (g)		% Absorption*	Frying time (min.)	Sensory evaluation		
	Before	After			Aroma	Color	Greasiness of crumb
a. Corn oil 163°C							
177°C							
190°C							
204°C							
b. Peanut oil 163°C							
177°C							
190°C							
204°C							
c. Shortening 163°C							
177°C							
190°C							
204°C							

$^*\dfrac{\text{final weight} - \text{original weight}}{\text{original weight}} \times 100 = \%$ fat absorption

Name

ADDITIONAL OBSERVATIONS AND NOTES

CHART 4.2.2   FAT ABSORPTION AND DEEP FAT FRYING OF DOUGHNUTS (*CONTINUED*)

Treatment	Weight (g)		% Absorption*	Frying time (min.)	Sensory evaluation		
	Before	After			Aroma	Color	Greasiness of crumb
d. Old oil 163°C							
177°C							
190°C							
204°C							
e. Old and new oil 163°C							
177°C							
190°C							
204°C							

$$\frac{\text{*final weight } - \text{ original weight}}{\text{original weight}} \times 100 = \% \text{ fat absorption}$$

Name

ADDITIONAL OBSERVATIONS AND NOTES

CHART 4.2.3   FLOW PROPERTIES OF SELECTED OILS

Type	Flow time (sec)		Appearance	
	Before frying	**After frying**	**Before frying**	**After frying**
a. Corn oil				
b. Peanut oil				
c. Shortening				
d. Old oil				
e. 1/2 old, 1/2 fresh oil				

ADDITIONAL OBSERVATIONS AND NOTES

EVALUATION

1. Compare the smoke points obtained from heating fresh fats and oils. For samples that are either unusually low or high, see the table of ingredients (Chart 4.1.1) to explain the variations.

2. Calculate the percent fat absorption as follows:

$$\% \text{ fat absorption} = \frac{\text{final weight} - \text{original weight}}{\text{original weight}} \times 100$$

Compare the absorption in the different frying media and at the different frying temperatures. Also compare the length of time required to brown the doughnuts to the same end point. Subjective evaluation should be directed toward the relative greasiness of the crumb, the aroma of the doughnut, and color. Note any differences in the flow properties of comparable fresh and used oils, as measured by timing the flow of 50 ml of **cool** oil before and after frying the doughnuts. Note any differences in color and odor that may be apparent.

STUDY QUESTIONS

1. Which fat had the highest smoke point? Which oil had the highest smoke point? Why did these results occur?

2. Would diet margarine be a suitable choice for frying doughnuts? Explain.

3. Explain the chemistry that is occurring when a fat is smoking.

4. Was there any difference in the fat absorption that occurred at the three temperatures used for frying? If so, what temperature resulted in the least absorption? Why?

5. Did the use of old oil influence the (a) absorption of fat, (b) aroma, (c) color of the food fried in it? How?

6. Which of the fats and oils tested in the deep fat frying experiment gave the best results? Why?

EXPERIMENT 4.3—FATS IN PASTRY
OBJECTIVES

Upon completion of the experiment, you will be able to:

1. Define flakiness in pastry and the factors contributing to this characteristic.
2. Operate the shortometer and explain how it measures tenderness in foods.
3. Explain the contradictions of tenderness and flakiness in pastry.
4. Evaluate pastries to discriminate between the qualities created by the use of the various fats tested.
5. Describe the characteristics in pastry that are promoted by various levels of fats in pastry.

BASIC FORMULA—PASTRY

1.5 g (1/4 tsp)	Salt
87 g (3/4 c)	All purpose flour
47 g (1/4 c)	Fat (shortening)
29.5 ml (2 tbsp)	Water

Add salt to flour and stir briefly with a 4-tined fork. Add the fat all at once. Use a pastry blender to cut in the fat until the pieces are about the size of uncooked rice grains. Sprinkle the water over the surface of the mixture, a drop at a time, while flipping the mixture upward lightly with a 4-tined fork. Continue sprinkling and flipping until all of the water has been added. With the fork, mash the dough together to make a ball of dough. This will take approximately 10 strokes. Do this as efficiently as possible, avoiding extra manipulation. When the dough forms a ball, turn the ball out onto a piece of wax paper about 12″ long. Very quickly manipulate the dough in the wax paper to form a more cohesive ball. Avoid holding the dough any longer than necessary to keep the dough as cool as possible.

Cut 2 strips of wax paper to fit the length and width between the guides on the special pastry board. Arrange one strip of wax paper on the special pastry board between the rolling guides. Place the dough on that strip of wax paper and quickly shape it into a flattened oblong shape to facilitate rolling the strip of dough. Place the other strip of wax paper over the dough. Lightly roll the dough until it is the thickness of the guides. If any of the dough squeezes out onto the guides, take it off with a knife and add it to the end of the strip of dough being rolled. Be sure no dough is on the guides when rolling is finished. This is important so that the thickness of the dough is controlled. Remove the top piece of wax paper, and cut dough rectangles efficiently with the rectangular cutter. Invert a cookie sheet over the pastry board, and quickly flip the sheet and board so that the rectangles of dough are on the cookie sheet. Remove the wax paper strip and the dough between the rectangles. Prick the surface of all of the rectangles with a fork to avoid blistering during baking. Bake at 218°C (425°F) until a pleasing, golden brown. Note the total baking time required.

PROCEDURE

1. **Type of fat**—Prepare the basic formula, but use the type of fat indicated below. These samples have a ratio of flour to fat of 3:1 (based on volume).

   a. *Shortening*—Prepare the basic formula using 47 g shortening.

   b. *Lard*—Prepare the basic formula using 47 g lard.

   c. *Margarine*—Prepare the basic formula using 47 g regular margarine.

   d. *Butter*—Prepare the basic formula using 47 g butter.

   e. *Oil*—Prepare the basic formula, but substitute 45 ml salad oil for the shortening.

   f. *Benecol*®—Prepare the basic formula using 47 g Benecol® for fat.

   g. *Take Control*®—Prepare the basic formula using 47 g Take Control® for fat.

2. **Amount of fat**—Prepare the basic formula, but use the amounts of fat indicated below. The first group has a ratio of flour to fat of 2:1, the second, 4:1.

   a. *Shortening, 2:1*—Use 70 g shortening in the basic formula.

   b. *Oil, 2:1*—Use 60 ml oil for fat in the basic formula.

   c. *Benecol*®, *2:1*—Prepare the basic formula using 70 g Benecol® for fat.

   d. *Take Control*®, *2:1*—Prepare the basic formula using 70 g Take Control® for fat.

   e. *Shortening, 4:1*—Prepare the basic formula using 35 g shortening for the fat.

   f. *Oil, 4:1*—Prepare the basic formula using 30 ml oil for the fat.

   g. *Benecol*®, *4:1*—Prepare the basic formula using 35 g Benecol® for the fat.

   h. *Take Control*®, *4:1*—Prepare the basic formula using 35 g Take Control® for the fat.

3. **Temperature of the fat**—The fats used in this section should be stored in the refrigerator for at least 12 hours prior to their use. Remove from the refrigerator, place in the freezer for 15 minutes. Weigh out the amount of fat needed for the experiment and return it to the freezer until it is needed in the experiment. Repeat procedure 1, but use the assigned chilled fat to make the pastry.

   a. *Shortening*—Prepare the basic formula pastry using 47 g chilled butter.

   b. *Lard*—Prepare the basic formula pastry using 47 g chilled lard.

   c. *Margarine*—Prepare the basic formula using 47 g chilled margarine.

   d. *Butter*—Prepare the basic formula pastry using 47 g chilled butter.

4. **Varying water and fat: butter/margarine pastries**—Make the following adjustments to determine the effectiveness of modifying butter or margarine quantities and compensating for their water content.

   a. *Equivalent of 3:1 ratio, butter*—Follow the basic formula, but use 57 g butter and 17 ml water.

   b. *Equivalent of 2:1 ratio, butter*—Prepare the basic formula, but use a total of 84 g butter and 13 ml water.

   c. *Equivalent of 4:1 ratio, butter*—Prepare the basic formula, but use 44 g butter and 20.5 ml water.

   d. *Equivalent of 3:1 ratio, margarine*—Prepare the basic formula, but use 57 g margarine and 17 ml water.

   e. *Equivalent of 2:1 ratio, margarine*—Prepare the basic formula, but use 84 g margarine and 13 ml water.

   f. *Equivalent of 4:1 ratio, margarine*—Prepare the basic formula, but use 44 g margarine and 20.5 ml water.

EVALUATION

Objective Evaluation   Flakiness can be determined by precisely measuring the height (in mm) of a stack of 3 of the wafers. (Ruler is in Appendix B.)

Tenderness is evaluated by using a shortometer. The shortometer is operated by checking to be sure both needles on the dial are in the correct 0 position, placing a sample across the bars on the shortometer, and then beginning the descent of the break bar. The descending bar is stopped as soon as the sample snaps, and the value on the dial is read and recorded. At least 3 samples of each type of pastry should be tested, and the mean of the 3 should be calculated.

Subjective evaluation   Subjective evaluation should include an assessment of the external appearance of the pastry, noting particularly the color and extent of blistering. To evaluate the interior, break the pastry and carefully examine the cross section to observe the flakiness of the pastry. Is the texture uniform and compact, or is it flaky? If it is flaky, determine whether there are many small compartments or whether there are a few large holes within the structure. Flavor should be judged carefully. This can best be done by taking a small bite of the pastry, assessing its flavor while it is in the mouth, and then exhaling after the bite has been swallowed. Aftertaste can be an important part of assessing flavor characteristics, and that is detected by exhaling through the nose to draw the flavor components into the nose. Tenderness can be evaluated by counting the number of chews.

STUDY QUESTIONS

1. Compare the fat and water content of butter, margarine, Benecol®, Take Control®, lard, and shortening. How does the composition of fats influence the formula to be used for pastry when fat substitutions are made?

CHART 4.3   EFFECT OF VARIATIONS IN FATS ON PASTRY

Treatment	Objective		Subjective				
	Short-ometer (g)	Height 3 wafers (mm)	Surface	Color	Texture	Flavor	(# Chews)
1. Type							
a. Shortening, 3:1							
b. Lard, 3:1							
c. Margarine, 3:1							
d. Butter, 3:1							
e. Oil, 3:1							
f. Benecol®, 3:1							
g. Take Control®, 3:1							
2. Amount							
a. Shortening, 2:1							
b. Oil, 2:1							
c. Benecol®, 2:1							
d. Take Control®, 2:1							
e. Shortening, 4:1							
f. Oil, 4:1							
g. Benecol®, 4:1							
h. Take Control®, 4:1							
3. Refrigerator Temperature a. Shortening, 3:1							
b. Lard, 3:1							
c. Margarine, 3:1							
d. Butter, 3:1							
4. Water and fat a. Butter, 3:1							
b. Butter, 2:1							
c. Butter, 4:1							
d. Margarine, 3:1							
e. Margarine, 2:1							
f. Margarine, 4:1							

Name

ADDITIONAL OBSERVATIONS AND NOTES

2. What is the interrelationship between flakiness and tenderness? Which fat gave the pastry that was most flaky? Which the least flaky?

3. Is there any apparent difference in the tenderness in pastry made with different fats? If so, which is the most tender? Which is the least tender? Why?

4. Is it possible to make a satisfactory pastry using: (a) butter; (b) margarine? If so, what changes should be recommended from the standard pastry formula? What are possible advantages to using butter in pastry? To using margarine?

5. Outline the procedure for operating the shortometer. What precautions need to be taken to ensure reliable results?

6. What are the advantages and disadvantages of each of the levels of fat tested? Which fat and at which ratio gave the best pastry? Explain why you chose that pastry.

7. Is there an advantage in chilling fat when making pastry? A disadvantage?

EXPERIMENT 4.4—FLAVOR AND EMULSIFICATION OF OILS
OBJECTIVES

Upon completion of the experiment, you will be able to:

1. Explain the theory of emulsion formation and the role of various emulsifying agents.
2. Characterize the flavor of the oils tested and evaluate potential uses of these substances on the basis of their flavor contributions.
3. Outline the changes that take place in an oil-in-water emulsion with increasing levels of oil. Explain how to re-establish a broken emulsion.

BASIC FORMULA—FLAVOR AND EMULSIFICATION OF OILS

17 g (1)	Egg yolk
15 ml (1 tbsp)	Vinegar
2 g (1/2 tsp)	Sugar
1.5 g (1/4 tsp)	Salt
0.6 g (1/4 tsp)	Dry mustard
0.6 g (1/4 tsp)	Paprika
118 ml (1/2 c)	Oil

Place the egg yolk, vinegar, and seasonings in a small bowl. Beat briefly with a rotary beater. Begin adding the oil, approximately 3 ml at a time. Beat slowly with the rotary beater after each addition until no trace of oil shows. Continue adding in very small additions until approximately 25 ml of oil have been added. Then the oil can be added more rapidly. One person can pour the oil while another beats the emulsion. Continue in this fashion until all the oil has been added.

PROCEDURE

1. **Type of oil**—Prepare the following mayonnaises using the type of oil indicated. Follow the basic formula.

   a. *Olive oil*—Prepare the basic formula using olive oil.

   b. *Soybean oil*—Prepare the basic formula using soybean oil.

   c. *Corn oil*—Prepare the basic formula using corn oil.

   d. *Cottonseed oil*—Prepare the basic formula using cottonseed oil.

   e. *Safflower oil*—Prepare the basic formula using safflower oil.

   f. *Sunflower oil*—Prepare the basic formula using sunflower oil.

   g. *Peanut oil*—Prepare the basic formula using peanut oil.

   h. *Canola oil*—Prepare the basic formula using canola oil.

2. **Variations**

   a. *Electric mixer*—Prepare the basic formula using corn oil and mixing on the slow speed of the electric mixer.

   b. *Increased oil*—Prepare the basic formula using corn oil, but add corn oil until no more can be added. If the emulsion breaks, put an egg yolk in a small bowl and gradually add the broken emulsion to the egg yolk while beating, as was done when the oil was added originally. Be sure to measure the total amount of oil that was added to the mayonnaise before the emulsion broke.

   c. *Red dye*—Stir 1 drop of red food coloring into a teaspoon of the corn oil mayonnaise made in 1c. Continue to stir until the color is uniform throughout the sample.

EVALUATION

Objective evaluation Depending on the size of the centrifuge tubes, pour equal amounts of all mayonnaise samples from 1 and 2a into the tubes (each labeled with the variation). Load the samples into the centrifuge, being sure that the centrifuge is balanced by having equal amounts across from each other. Centrifuge at the fastest setting for 15 seconds. Check to see which emulsions have broken, and remove them from the centrifuge. Determine the amount of oil that has separated in the broken emulsions. Reload the centrifuge to keep balanced with samples opposite each other, and then centrifuge another 15 seconds. Again, remove broken emulsions, measure the volume of separated oil, reload the centrifuge, and continue the cycle until all emulsions have broken. Freeze small samples of each mayonnaise and check the stability of the emulsion after thawing samples at the next laboratory session.

Subjective evaluation Subjective evaluation of mayonnaise is a useful means of identifying the flavor characteristics of the various oils used in this experiment. If the mayonnaises seem too oily to be palatable to sample, the sample can be placed on a corner of a soda cracker for evaluation.

CHART 4.4   FLAVOR AND STABILITY OF EMULSION

Treatment	Objective					Subjective		
	Time to break (sec.)	Amt. oil separated (ml)	Stability after freezing	Line Spread Fresh (mm)	Line Spread Stored (mm)	Color and Oiliness	Flavor	Mouthfeel
1. Type of Oil a. Olive								
b. Soybean								
c. Corn								
d. Cottonseed								
e. Safflower								
f. Sunflower								
g. Peanut								
h. Canola								
2. Variations a. Electric mixer								
b. Extra oil ____ ml oil								

Red dye (sketch here):

ADDITIONAL OBSERVATIONS AND NOTES

Evaluation should be directed toward appearance, including any suggestion of oiliness on the surface, and the color of the sample. Flavor and mouthfeel also are meaningful subjective evaluation criteria. Slice the sample with excess oil and observe the cut surface.

Microscopic examination   Place a drop of the emulsion containing the red dye (2c) on a slide. View the emulsion under the microscope and sketch the appearance. Since the red food coloring is water soluble, the areas tinted with the dye will be the vinegar, and the oil will be untinted.

STUDY QUESTIONS

1. Define an emulsion. What is the difference between an oil-in-water and a water-in-oil emulsion? What type of emulsion is mayonnaise? Does the microscope slide confirm your classification?

2. What is the role of dry ingredients in mayonnaise? Of egg yolk?

3. Is there any difference in the stability of mayonnaise when different oils are used? If so, which is the most stable? Which is least stable? Why is this so?

4. Describe the flavor of each of the mayonnaise samples. Which oil is in the most acceptable mayonnaise? Which oil is in the least acceptable sample?

5. How can a broken oil-in-water emulsion be re-established?

6. Does freezing influence stability of mayonnaise? Why?

5

Dairy Products

Dairy products present challenges and opportunities when making a range of food products; examples include acid and enzyme (rennin) coagulation of milk proteins. Coagulation of casein is useful in making cheeses and certain clotted milk products, but it may be confounding when attempting to prepare milk-containing dishes of high quality. Dairy products have roles to perform in recipes utilizing milk or cream foams. These foams may be stabilized by the presence of fat or by a concentration of milk proteins.

In this chapter, the experiments will demonstrate the merits of various milk, cheese, and cream products available today. Cow's milk products include whole, reduced fat, low fat, and fat free (nonfat) homogenized fluid milk products that have all been pasteurized for safety. Other pasteurized cow's milk products include lactase-containing milks of varying fat content, buttermilk, canned evaporated milks ranging in fat levels from whole to nonfat, canned sweetened condensed milk, sterilized milk for storage at room temperature until opened, dried milk solids, and imitation milks. Goat's milk and soy milk are milk alternatives of particular importance for people allergic to cow's milk.

The cooking characteristics of natural and processed cheeses made from goat's, sheep's and cow's milk are compared in these experiments. Cream products tested in this chapter include half and half (12% fat), light cream (20% fat), and whipping cream (35% fat), as well as refrigerated and frozen stabilized whipped cream or imitation products.

The technological advances in dairy products are extensive. This chapter discusses new products as well as traditional dairy foods.

EXPERIMENT 5.1—COAGULATION OF MILK
OBJECTIVES

Upon completion of the experiment, you will be able to:

1. Explain the change in solubility that occurs in milk protein as the medium approaches the isoelectric point.
2. Explain the role of salts in coagulating milk proteins.
3. Outline ways of minimizing coagulation when this change would be detrimental to the quality of milk-containing products.
4. Compare the flavor, cost, convenience, and cooking applications of various types of milks and sour cream available to consumers today.

PROCEDURE

Perform the tests below on the milk assigned from the following milks: (a) whole milk, (b) reduced fat milk, (c) low fat milk, (d) fat free milk, (e) buttermilk, (f) Lactaid®, (g) nonfat dried milk (reconstituted), (h) evaporated whole milk (reconstituted), (i) sweetened condensed milk, (j) goat's milk, and (k) soy milk.

1. **Type of milk**—Label a glass for each type of milk and pour 115 ml of each type of milk (reconstituted if evaporated or dried) into the appropriate glass. Cover with plastic wrap and refrigerate until ready for evaluation.

2. **Effect of salts**—Dice a cube of ham and place in a custard cup with 50 ml fluid milk. Check the pH of the milk. Label the type of milk on the custard cup and place in a pan with the other labeled cups. Place pan on the oven rack and quickly, but carefully, pour boiling water into the pan until the water rises around the cups to about the level of the milk. Bake at 350°F (177°C) for 1 hour. Remove cups from water and cool at room temperature. Check the pH after the milk has cooled.

3. **Effect of acid**

   3.1. **Variations in milk**—Combine 15 ml vinegar with 100 ml of the assigned milk. Stir well. Measure the pH. Let stand 5 minutes or longer before observing the results.

   3.2. **Method of combining ingredients**—Using this basic formula, prepare a sauce by each of the 3 methods outlined below.

BASIC FORMULA—COMBINING INGREDIENTS

7 g (1/2 tbsp)	Margarine
3.5 g (1/2 tbsp)	Flour
1 g (1/6 tsp)	Salt
60 ml (1/4 c)	Milk
60 ml; (1/4 c)	Tomato juice
2.5 ml (1/2 tsp)	Lemon juice

Melt margarine. Stir in flour and salt to make a smooth paste. Gradually stir in the milk to make a slurry. Slowly stir in the two juices. Measure pH. Quickly heat to boiling while stirring constantly with a wooden spoon. Cool the sample and measure the pH.

a. *Hot juice to milk sauce*—Proceed as in the basic formula, but heat the tomato and lemon juices before stirring into the milk slurry. Heat to boiling and serve.

b. *Hot tomato sauce added to cold milk*—Melt the margarine. Stir in flour and salt to make a smooth paste. Stir in two juices. Heat with stirring to make hot paste. Stir into cold milk. Heat to boiling while stirring.

c. *Hot tomato sauce to hot milk*—Melt the margarine. Stir in flour and salt to make smooth paste. Stir in the two juices. Heat with stirring to make hot paste. Stir into hot milk. Heat with stirring until mixture boils.

4. **Effect of type of sour cream**
   a. *Sour cream*—Follow the basic formula, using dairy sour cream.
   b. *Light sour cream*—Follow the basic formula, using light sour cream.
   c. *Nonfat sour cream*—Follow the basic formula, using nonfat sour cream.
   d. *Imitation sour cream*—Follow the basic formula, using imitation sour cream.

BASIC FORMULA—EFFECT OF SOUR CREAM

Measure the pH of the assigned sour cream. Place 250 g of the assigned sour cream in a 400 ml beaker; heat in a water bath maintained at 90°C. Stir sour cream with a 4-tined fork at the rate of 10 strokes per minute. Note the time required to heat the sour cream until it curdles. Put the curdled sour cream and its package on the display table.

EVALUATION

1. For the fluid chilled milks, subjective evaluation should focus on flavor qualities, mouthfeel, and general palatability. Compare possible uses and relative costs.

2. Use a spoon to determine the relative smoothness of the milks cooked with ham.

3. Note the pH and consistency of acidified milks. To evaluate the tomato soups, examine them visually for any evidence of curdling. Note also the presence of lumps due to non-uniform gelatinization of the starch. Curdling will result in a somewhat modified appearance, whereas improper gelatinization will show some distinct lumps of white starch.

4. Examine the curdled sour creams to determine the comparative curd size, viscosity, and separation.

STUDY QUESTIONS

1. Compare the advantages and disadvantages of the various fluid milks that were sampled as chilled liquid. Cite an example when each of the milks might be a particularly suitable choice for a consumer.

2. Does heating result in a change in the pH of milk over a period of time? If so, what implications does this have for writing procedures for recipes utilizing milk in cooking?

3. Explain the curdling that may happen when ham and other salt-containing foods are heated with milk. Explain the curdling that occurs after acid is added to milk. Did all of the milks behave exactly the same?

4. Define isoelectric point. What pH is the isoelectric point of casein? What is the approximate pH of tomato juice? What was the pH of the milk used in the experiment?

5. Why is the addition of tomato juice to milk less likely to cause curdling than when milk is added to the tomato juice?

6. Can any of the reduced fat or imitation sour cream be substituted satisfactorily for sour cream in a product such as beef stroganoff? Explain your answer.

CHART 5.1.1   FLUID MILKS EVALUATION

Type	Cost/cup	Aroma	Color	Flavor	Mouthfeel	Palatability
1. **Fluid (homo.)** a. Whole						
b. Reduced fat						
c. Low fat						
d. Fat free						
e. Buttermilk						
f. Lactaid®						
g. Nonfat dried						
h. Evaporated, whole						
i. Sweetened condensed						
j. Goat's						
k. Soy milk						

Name

ADDITIONAL OBSERVATIONS AND NOTES

CHART 5.1.2   EFFECTS OF SALTS

Type of milk	pH of milk		Appearance after cooking
	Before	**After**	
1. Fluid (homo.) a. Whole			
b. Reduced fat			
c. Fat free			
d. Buttermilk			
e. Lactaid®			
f. Nonfat dried			
2. Canned a. Evap., whole			
b. Evap., low fat			
c. Evap., nonfat			
d. Sweetened condensed			
3. Goat's			
4. Soy milk			

Name

ADDITIONAL OBSERVATIONS AND NOTES

CHART 5.1.3.1   EFFECT OF ACID

Type of milk	pH of acidified milk	Consistency after 5 min.
a. Whole		
b. Reduced fat		
c. Low fat		
d. Fat free		
e. Buttermilk		
f. Lactaid®		
g. Nonfat dried		
h. Evaporated whole		
i. Sweetened condensed		
j. Goat's		
k. Soy		

CHART 5.1.3.2   EFFECT OF ACID (CONTINUED)

Method	pH		Appearance
	Before cooking	After cooking	
a. Hot juice to milk			
b. Hot sauce to cold milk			
c. Hot tomato to hot milk			

Name

ADDITIONAL OBSERVATIONS AND NOTES

CHART 5.1.4 EFFECT OF TYPE OF SOUR CREAM

Type	pH	Curdling time (min.)	Appearance
a. Sour cream			
b. Light sour cream			
c. Nonfat sour cream			
d. Imitation sour cream			

ADDITIONAL OBSERVATIONS AND NOTES

EXPERIMENT 5.2—CLOTTING OF MILK
OBJECTIVES

Upon completion of the experiment, you will be able to:

1. Outline the basic method for clotting milk with rennin.
2. Explain the clotting of milk that occurs in the preparation of yogurt.
3. Describe the changes that occur in milk when acid or enzyme is added.
4. Describe the browning reaction and explain why this can be seen so graphically when sweetened condensed milk is heated.
5. Define curd and whey and explain how they are utilized in food products.

BASIC FORMULA—COTTAGE CHEESE

472 ml	Milk
1 tablet	Rennet

Dissolve rennet in 1 tablespoon of lukewarm water while milk is being heated to 37°C. Add rennet and let stand 1 hour. Use a knife to slice curd into 1/2-inch cubes. Reheat to 37°C and maintain that temperature until whey separates. Transfer the clotted mixture to a sieve lined with a double layer of cheesecloth. Collect the whey in a beaker below the sieve. Measure the volume of whey in a graduated cylinder. Place the curd in a serving dish for evaluation.

PROCEDURE

1. **Cottage Cheese**—Using the basic formula above, prepare cottage cheese and whey from each of the following milks:

   a. *Fat free milk*

   b. *Fat free milk, 2x rennet*—Double the rennet to 2 tablets.

   c. *Homogenized whole milk*

   d. *Nonfat dry milk*—Use 45.4 g nonfat dry milk solids and 442.5 ml water.

   e. *Evaporated fat free milk*—Use undiluted.

   f. *Evaporated fat free milk, diluted*—Use 236 ml milk plus 236 ml water.

BASIC FORMULA—YOGURT

472 ml	Milk
51 g	Yogurt (unflavored)

Heat the milk to 49°C. Stir 50 ml of the warmed milk into the yogurt and then return the yogurt mixture to the pan of warm milk. Maintain the milk-yogurt mixture at 47°C for 6 to 8 hours. This may be done by placing the pan (covered with aluminum foil) in a gas oven heated only by the pilot light. Refrigerate at least 4 hours after the product thickens before evaluating the samples.

---

2. **Yogurt**—Using the basic formula above, prepare yogurt from each of the following milks:

   a. *Fat free milk*—Prepare the basic formula using fat free milk.

   b. *Homogenized whole milk*—Prepare the basic formula using homogenized whole milk.

   c. *Homogenized whole milk + solids*—Add 17 g nonfat dry milk solids to homogenized whole milk. Prepare the basic formula with this milk preparation.

   d. *Nonfat dry milk*—Combine 45.4 g nonfat dry milk solids and 442.5 ml water. Prepare the basic formula with this reconstituted milk.

   e. *Evaporated whole milk (undiluted)*—Prepare the basic formula using undiluted evaporated whole milk.

   f. *Evaporated whole milk (diluted)*—Combine 236 ml whole evaporated milk with 236 ml water. Prepare the basic formula with this diluted evaporated whole milk.

   g. *Evaporated fat free milk (undiluted)*—Prepare the basic formula using undiluted evaporated fat free milk.

   h. *Evaporated fat free milk (diluted)*—Combine 236 ml evaporated fat free milk and 236 ml water. Prepare the basic formula using this diluted evaporated fat free milk.

3. **Reactions with acid**—Stir 5 ml lemon juice into 20 ml milk. Let stand at least 15 minutes before noting the results. Use the following milks:

   a. *Evaporated whole milk (undiluted)*

   b. *Sweetened condensed milk (undiluted)*

   c. *Sweetened condensed fat free milk (undiluted)*

4. **Reactions with heat**—Using the type of milk assigned, heat 10 test tubes (each containing 20 ml milk) in a boiling water bath. The level of the water should be maintained at approximately the height of the

milk in the test tubes. Remove 1 test tube at each of the following times: 10, 20, 30, 40, 50, 60, 75, 90, 105, and 120 minutes. Be sure to label each sample before setting it aside for evaluation.

   a. *Evaporated whole milk (undiluted)*

   b. *Sweetened condensed milk (undiluted)*

EVALUATION

1. Cottage cheese in this experiment is evaluated subjectively, noting particularly the flavor and tenderness of the curd. If desired, salt may be added to the curd to enhance the flavor. The volume and flavor of the whey also should be noted.

2. Yogurt is evaluated subjectively. Note particuarly the tenderness of the gel, the flavor, and the amount of syneresis.

3. Compare the viscosity of the evaporated and sweetened condensed milks to which lemon juice has been added. Note the comparative smoothness of the two products.

4. Evaluate the heated evaporated and sweetened condensed milk products by noting specifically the color changes that may be discernible and also noting viscosity at each time interval.

STUDY QUESTIONS

1. What is rennin? Describe its effect on milk. Why does too high a temperature interfere with the action of rennin?

2. Describe the method used for making cottage cheese with rennin. Explain any precautions that are included in the procedure. Explain why the curd is cut.

3. What nutrients are found in the whey from rennin-coagulated milk? From acid-coagulated milk? Identify uses for whey.

4. Describe the changes that take place during the preparation of yogurt.

5. Compare the changes when acid was added to evaporated milk and to sweetened condensed milk. Why do these changes occur?

6. Compare the changes observed as the evaporated and sweetened condensed milk were heated. What reaction primarily causes the color change?

7. Can evaporated milk and sweetened condensed milk be used interchangeably in recipes? Explain your answer.

8. Which milks are best for making cottage cheese? Which are not well suited to making cottage cheese? Explain your recommendations.

9. Which milks are best suited to making yogurt? Which are not well suited to making yogurt? Explain your recommendations.

CHART 5.2.1   COTTAGE CHEESE

Type of milk	Whey		Curd	
	Volume	**Flavor**	**Flavor**	**Tenderness**
a. Fat free milk				
b. Fat free milk, double enzyme				
c. Homogenized whole milk				
d. Nonfat dry milk solids (reconstituted)				
e. Evaporated fat free milk (undiluted)				
f. Evaporated fat free milk (diluted)				

Name

ADDITIONAL OBSERVATIONS AND NOTES

CHART 5.2.2   YOGURT

Type of milk	Tenderness of gel	Flavor	Syneresis
a. Fat free milk			
b. Homo. whole milk			
c. Homo. whole + nonfat dry solids			
d. Nonfat dry milk (diluted)			
e. Evaporated whole milk (undiluted)			
f. Evaporated whole milk (diluted)			
g. Evaporated fat free milk (undiluted)			
h. Evaporated fat free milk (diluted)			

Name

ADDITIONAL OBSERVATIONS AND NOTES

CHART 5.2.3   REACTIONS WITH ACID

Treatment	Relative viscosity	Consistency
1.a. Evaporated whole milk		
1.b. Sweetened condensed whole milk		
1.c. Sweetened condensed fat free milk		

Name

ADDITIONAL OBSERVATIONS AND NOTES

CHART 5.2.4   REACTIONS WITH HEAT

Treatment	Color	Viscosity	Flavor
2.a. Evaporated milk 10 min.			
20 min.			
30 min.			
40 min.			
50 min.			
60 min.			
75 min.			
90 min.			
105 min.			
120 min.			
2.b. Sweetened condensed milk 10 min.			
20 min.			
30 min.			
40 min.			
50 min.			
60 min.			
75 min.			
90 min.			
105 min.			
120 min.			

Name

ADDITIONAL OBSERVATIONS AND NOTES

EXPERIMENT 5.3—FOAMS
OBJECTIVES

Upon completion of the experiment, you will be able to:

1. Outline the role of protein in foam formation.
2. Outline the role of fat in foam formation.
3. Explain the effect of varying the following factors in a foam:
   a. Fat content
   b. Protein content
   c. Temperature
   d. pH
   e. Stabilizer (gelatin)
   f. Extent of beating
4. Outline the best method for making a foam using (a) nonfat dry milk solids, (b) evaporated milk, and (c) whipping cream.
5. Explain the change that occurs when whipping cream is beaten too long.
6. Interpret the effects of freezing and thawing dairy product foams.

BASIC FORMULA—FOAM

118 ml   Milk or Cream

Using the conditions described below, whip the assigned milk or cream (118 ml) with an electric mixer at high speed until the foam is as stiff as possible (maximum of 15 minutes) or until it piles well. Note the time required for forming the foam. Transfer the foam to a funnel lined with a layer of filter paper and use a ring stand to hold the funnel above a graduated cylinder. Use a skewer to measure the vertical height of the foam. Collect the filtrate for a total of 1 hour, noting the volume after 10 minutes, 20 minutes, 30, and 60 minutes. Evaluate the appearance of the foam after 1 hour.

PROCEDURE

1. **Evaporated milk**

   a. *Chill, undiluted*—Chill undiluted evaporated whole milk in a freezer tray in the freezer until ice crystals form around the edge. Then whip on the fast speed of an electric mixer, according to the basic formula.

   b. *Room temperature, undiluted*—Whip undiluted evaporated milk at room temperature. Whip on the fast speed of the electric mixer, as described in the basic formula.

   c. *Chill, undiluted, acid*—Chill undiluted evaporated whole milk as described in the basic formula, but add 5 ml lemon juice at the beginning of the beating period.

    d. *Chill, undiluted, gelatin*—Combine 1 envelope of gelatin with 60 ml water and heat in a boiling water bath until gelatin dissolves. Add 5 ml of the dissolved gelatin to undiluted evaporated milk. Chill in a freezer tray in the freezer until ice crystals form around the edge. Whip as described in the basic formula.

2. **Nonfat dry milk**

    a. *Milk/water, 1:1*—Reconstitute 30 g nonfat dry milk solids with 118 ml water. When thoroughly blended, measure 118 ml and whip as described above.

    b. *Milk/water, 2:1*—Reconstitute 60 g nonfat dry milk solids with 118 ml water. When thoroughly blended, measure 118 ml and whip as described above.

    c. *Milk/water, 1:2*—Reconstitute 15 g nonfat dry milk solids with 118 ml water. When thoroughly blended, measure 118 ml and whip as described above.

    d. *Milk/water, 1:1, lemon*—Reconstitute 30 g nonfat dry milk solids with 118 ml water. When thoroughly blended, measure 113 ml of the reconstituted milk and add 5 ml lemon juice. Whip as described above.

    e. *Milk/water, 1:1, gelatin*—Reconstitute 30 g nonfat dry milk solids with 118 ml water. When thoroughly blended, measure 118 ml of the reconstituted milk and 5 ml of the room temperature gelatin blend (prepared in 1d). Whip as described above.

3. **Cream**—Follow the basic formula to prepare foams for the following variations:

    a. *Half and half, room temperature*

    b. *Half and half, refrigerator temperature*

    c. *Coffee cream, room temperature*

    d. *Coffee cream, refrigerator temperature*

    e. *Light whipping cream, room temperature*

    f. *Light whipping cream, refrigerator temperature*

    g. *Heavy whipping cream, room temperature*

    h. *Heavy whipping cream, refrigerator temperature*

    i. *Heavy whipping cream, refrigerator temperature, sugar*—Heavy whipping cream at refrigerator temperature and with 25 g sugar folded in after the foam is completed.

    j. *Heavy whipping cream, refrigerator temperature, over-whipped*—Heavy whipping cream at refrigerator temperature, but whipped until the emulsion reverses and butter begins to form. Press out the liquid to form butter. Add salt to taste, if desired. Do not attempt to drain this in a funnel.

k. *Non-dairy whipping cream, refrigerator temperature*

l. *Aerosol and tub whipped creams*—Place whipped heavy cream (aerosol) in a funnel and proceed according to the measurements described in the basic formula. Place whipped heavy cream (tub) in a funnel and proceed according to the measurements described in the basic formula.

EVALUATION

1. Compare the times required to form the various foams prepared in the series. Note also the relative volumes of the various products when the foam is first formed and the relative stability of the foams. The volume of the filtrate is a direct indicator of the instability of the foams. Note also the texture of the foams and any differences in mouthfeel.

2. Compare the texture of the cream foams with the evaporated milk foams. Also compare stability. Calculate the nutritive values of these foams, using label information or a table of food composition. Compare the foams.

STUDY QUESTIONS

1. Why does increasing the concentration of protein increase the stability of a foam? Does increasing the fat content have a similar influence?

2. What is the effect of adding acid to a milk foam? Of adding gelatin? Explain the theory behind the action of each. Would these same additions have similar effects on cream foams? Why?

3. What effect does temperature have upon the formation of milk foams? Of cream foams?

4. Contrast the probable effect of over-beating the milk foam with the effect of over-beating a cream foam.

5. Compare the nutritive merits of milk foams with those made with cream. Compare these products also with commercial foam products in aerosol and plastic containers. Compare the costs.

6. Outline the method preferred for making a stable foam using nonfat dry milk solids.

7. Outline the method preferred for making a stable foam using evaporated milk.

8. Outline the method preferred for making a stable foam using cream. What level of fat is needed to make a stable cream foam?

9. Discuss the theory of the change that results when cream is whipped and ultimately becomes butter.

CHART 5.3   EVAPORATED MILK FOAMS AND CREAM FOAMS

Treatment	Time (min.)	Height (cm)	ml of drainage (min) 10	20	30	60	Texture	Flavor	Mouth-feel
1. Evaporated milk foams a. Chill, not diluted									
b. Room temp., not diluted									
c. Chill, lemon juice									
d. Chill, gelatin									
2. Nonfat dry milk foams a. Milk/water, 1:1									
b. Milk/water, 2:1									
c. Milk/water, 1:2									
d. Milk/water, 1:1 plus lemon									
e. Milk/water, 1:1 plus gelatin									
3. Cream foams a. Half and half room temp.									
b. Half and half, chilled									
c. Coffee cream, room temp.									
d. Coffee cream, chilled									
e. Light whip. cream, room temp.									
f. Light whip. cream, chilled									
g. Heavy whip. cream, room temp.									
h. Heavy whip. cream, chilled									
i. Heavy whip. cream, chilled, sugar									
j. Heavy whip. cream, chilled, over-beaten (butter)			XXX	XXX	XXX	XXX			
k. Non-dairy whipping cream									
l. Whipped heavy cream (aerosol)	XXX								
cream (tub)	XXX								

Name

ADDITIONAL OBSERVATIONS AND NOTES

EXPERIMENT 5.4—CHEESE AND SOUR CREAM
OBJECTIVES

Upon completion of the experiment, you will be able to:

1. Identify some of the various types of cheese available to consumers today and discuss the rationale underlying the reasons for developing them.
2. Select cheeses well suited to use in products featuring melted cheese.
3. Select cheese and sour creams suited for use in dips.

BASIC FORMULA—HEATED CHEESE

2 circle cuts of cheese 3" diameter and 1/4" thick

Place one cheese slice on a plate for evaluation; put the label next to it on the display table. Place the other slice of cheese on a paper towel and carefully trace its pattern on the towel using a lead pencil with a sharp point. Place the cheese and its towel on a jelly roll pan. Heat in an oven preheated to 300°F (150°C). Precisely note the time required for the cheese to soften sufficiently to start to flow. Remove from the oven. Measure the diameter of the melted cheese at its widest point; measure the diameter at its narrowest point. Calculate the mean of the two diameters.

For evaluation, transfer the cheese to a sample plate, and place the paper towel on display next to the plate.

PROCEDURE

1. **Types of cheeses**—Using the assigned cheese, follow the basic formula above.

   a. *Swiss cheese*

   b. *Fat free Swiss cheese*

   c. *Monterey Jack cheese*

   d. *Reduced fat Monterey Jack cheese*

   e. *Fat free Monterey Jack cheese*

   f. *Tofu cheese alternative (Monterey Jack)*

   g. *Cheddar cheese*

   h. *Reduced fat cheddar cheese*

   i. *Tofu cheese alternative (cheddar)*

2. **Dip bases**—Using assigned cheese or sour cream, prepare the basic formula.

   a. *Cream cheese*

   b. *Light cream cheese*

   c. *Soft cream cheese*

BASIC FORMULA—DIP BASE

85 g Cream cheese
4 g Dry onion soup mix

Whip ingredients together for 2 minutes at high speed on a electric mixer.

---

d. *Fat free cream cheese*

e. *Sour cream*—Prepare basic formula substituting sour cream for cream cheese and stirring ingredients 50 strokes with a 4-tined fork. Do not use the electric mixer.

f. *Fat free sour cream*—Prepare as described in 2e, but use fat free sour cream in place of sour cream.

g. *Imitation sour cream*—Prepare as described in 2e, but use imitation sour cream in place of sour cream.

EVALUATION

Objective testing for the dip is done by using the penetrometer to measure viscosity. *Subjective testing* is done by dipping a piece of cracker into the dip and noting the ease of dipping, textural characteristics, and flavor.

STUDY QUESTIONS

1. Which ingredients were added to the reduced fat and fat free cheeses to compensate for the roles of fat in cheese cookery? Compare the melting characteristics of these cheeses with their full fat counterparts.

2. Are tofu cheeses as palatable as their comparable full fat cheeses? Describe similarities and differences. Who would be likely purchasers of tofu cheeses?

3. How does the fat level influence the characteristics of a dip made with cream cheese? With sour cream?

4. Identify the advantages and disadvantage of using cream cheese versus sour cream as the base for a dip.

CHART 5.4.1 HEATED CHEESES

Cheese	Appearance		Mean dia. (mm)	Flavor	# of chews
	Towel	Cheese			
a. Swiss					
b. Fat free Swiss					
c. Monterey Jack					
d. Reduced fat Monterey Jack					
e. Fat free Monterey Jack					
f. Tofu alternative (Monterey Jack)					
g. Cheddar					
h. Reduced fat Cheddar					
i. Tofu alternative (Cheddar)					

Name

ADDITIONAL OBSERVATIONS AND NOTES

CHART 5.4.2   DIP BASE

Dip base	Penetrometer (mm)	Ease of dipping	Texture	Flavor
a. Cream cheese				
b. Light cream cheese				
c. Soft cream cheese				
d. Fat free cream cheese				
e. Sour cream				
f. Fat free sour cream				
g. Imitation sour cream				

ADDITIONAL OBSERVATIONS AND NOTES

6
Meats, Fish, and Poultry

Meats, fish, and poultry command a large fraction of the food dollar. Therefore, knowledge of purchasing and preparation of these foods is of great importance to achieve the best possible results, whether feeding a large number of people or a small family.

The experiments in this chapter are structured to provide experience in working with meats, fish, poultry, and soy protein, and to illustrate the characteristics, advantages, and disadvantages accompanying their preparation and service. The effectiveness of various kinds of equipment (including the microwave oven, crock pot, and pressure saucepan) for preparing protein foods also will be illustrated in these experiments.

One important aspect of consumer acceptance of meats and meat alternatives is the tenderness of the item being judged. Changes in connective tissue and muscle proteins are accomplished by various cooking procedures. The use of enzymes is another means of modifying tenderness of protein-rich foods. The tenderizing effect of these various approaches is demonstrated in the experiments in this chapter.

Flavor and juiciness are two other important criteria for evaluating the preparation and quality of meat and meat substitutes. These characteristics are influenced by preparation techniques. Illustrations of factors modifying flavor and juiciness are included in this chapter.

Meat experiments present particular difficulties in securing samples that allow valid comparisons. As much as possible, samples should be from matched sides of an animal and be the same size. Careful records of weights before and after cooking are essential. Information on cooking times is vital to aid in interpreting results. The control of end points is done through the use of thermometers rather than clocks in these experiments. The somewhat variable rate of heat penetration from one cut to another makes final interior temperature a better guide than cooking times.

EXPERIMENT 6.1—SOY PROTEIN SUBSTITUTES
OBJECTIVES

Upon completion of the experiment, you will be able to:

1. Outline the benefits and disadvantages of using textured soy protein in ground meat formulas.
2. Describe the textural and flavor characteristics of textured soy protein.
3. Contrast the cooking characteristics of ground meat products containing varying levels of textured soy protein.

BASIC FORMULA–MEAT LOAF

454 g (1 lb)	Ground beef
48 g (1)	Egg
45 g (1/3 c)	Onion, chopped
2.5 g (1/2 tsp)	Salt

Weigh the empty loaf pan, and record the weight. Thoroughly stir the ingredients together. Shape into a loaf 3″ × 6″ and place in the loaf pan. Weigh and record the weight of the loaf pan plus the unbaked meat loaf. Place in an oven preheated to 325°F (163°C). Place an oven-proof thermometer in the meat loaf, being certain the bulb of the thermometer is in the center of the loaf. If necessary, use a rack positioned above the meat loaf to support the thermometer. Bake for approximately 60 minutes until the thermometer temperature reaches 77°C (170°F). Note the total baking time required to reach that temperature. Allow the loaf to cool for 5 minutes before weighing the pan and its contents. Remove the meat loaf and weigh it. Weigh the pan and the drippings that are in it. Calculate total cooking losses and drip loss. Pour the drippings into a graduated cylinder to cool. Record the milliliters of fat that have risen to the top after the drippings have cooled.

PROCEDURE

1. **Control**—Prepare the basic formula as described above.

2. **25% TSP**—Reconstitute 29 g of textured soy protein (TSP) with 87 ml water. Allow TSP to absorb water before combining the reconstituted TSP with 340 g ground beef; proceed to mix in the remaining ingredients and prepare as in the basic formula.

3. **50% TSP**—Reconstitute 57 g of TSP with 171 ml water. Allow TSP to absorb water before combining the reconstituted TSP with 227 g ground beef; proceed to mix in the remaining ingredients and prepare as in the basic formula.

4. **100% TSP**—Reconstitute 114 g TSP with 340 ml water. Allow TSP to absorb water before combining the reconstituted TSP with the egg, onion, and salt; proceed as in the basic formula.

EVALUATION

1. Calculations to determine total drip losses should be made for each of the variations. The baking time also should be computed. If the information is available, determine the costs and nutritive value of the variations.

2. Subjective evaluation is done by comparing general appearance, juiciness, flavor, and tenderness of the various samples. Tenderness can be evaluated by counting the number of chews. To do this, each judge needs to identify the precise area in the mouth where chewing will be done, the exact size of the bite, and the final endpoint for chewing. Scores by the same judge then can be compared for relative tenderness of the samples. Comparisons between number of chews by various judges are not made, but the relative rankings of the different variations determined by the judges can be compared.

STUDY QUESTIONS

1. What is the effect of increasing levels of TSP on:
   a. Tenderness?
   b. Juiciness?
   c. Appearance?
   d. Flavor?

2. How does the drip loss of 100% ground beef meat loaf compare with loaves containing 25%, 50%, and 100% TSP? Is there any relationship between fat loss and apparent juiciness?

3. At what maximum level would it be acceptable to incorporate TSP into ground meat products? What is the economic advantage at that level?

4. Identify the advantages and disadvantages of using TSP at various levels. Include nutritional considerations (see a nutrition text and/or food composition table to assist in answering this question).

5. Does TSP influence baking times? If so, how?

CHART 6.1   MEAT LOAVES

Characteristic	Treatment			
	1. 100% beef*	2. 25% TSP 75% beef	3. 50% TSP 50% beef	4. 100% TSP
Appearance				
Flavor				
Juiciness				
Tenderness (# chews)				
Baking time				
Drip loss[1]				
Fat loss[2]				
Total cooking loss[3]				
Cost				

*Control
[1]Drip loss (%) = [(wt. pan + drippings) − (wt. pan)]/(wt. raw meat) × 100 = _____ %
[2]Fat loss = amount measured in graduated cylinder
[3]Total loss (%) = (wt. unbaked loaf − wt. baked loaf)/wt. unbaked loaf × 100

Name

ADDITIONAL OBSERVATIONS AND NOTES

EXPERIMENT 6.2 MEAT COOKERY: EQUIPMENT VARIATIONS OBJECTIVES

Upon completion of the experiment, you will be able to:

1. Outline the procedures recommended for cooking less tender cuts of meat by the use of a slow cooker, pressure saucepan, microwave oven, and conventional braising technique.
2. Evaluate the merits of a marinade in tenderizing less tender cuts of meat.
3. Identify the advantages and disadvantages of cooking less tender cuts of meat in slow cookers, pressure saucepans, microwave ovens, and by braising in a Dutch oven.

BASIC FORMULA—BEEF STEW MEAT

~227g	Beef cubes (1″ on side)
200 ml	Liquid
1 g	Salt

(Record exact weight of meat)

Marinade (Procedures 3, 5, 7, and 9)

2	Onions, sliced
2 c	Red wine
1 1/2 c	Water

In a large covered casserole dish or Dutch oven, combine the wine and onions. Add 2 lb of beef stew meat and stir to blend. Let stand for an hour at room temperature or overnight in the refrigerator. Stir at least once while marinating the meat.

PROCEDURE

1. **Slow cooker (high heat)**—Follow the basic formula. Place the meat in the bottom of a slow cooker. Add 200 ml water and salt. Cover the pot and set on high setting. Cook covered for 4 hours.

2. **Slow cooker (low heat)**—Follow the basic formula. Place meat in the bottom of a slow cooker. Add 200 ml of water and salt. Cover the slow cooker and cook on low setting for 8 hours.

3. **Slow cooker (low heat, marinade)**—Follow the basic formula, using marinated beef. Place in slow cooker with 200 ml marinade and salt. Cover and cook on low setting 8 hours.

4. **Pressure saucepan (no marinade)**—Prepare according to the basic formula. Follow the directions for the pressure saucepan being used. Place the weighed meat and 200 ml water plus salt in the pressure saucepan. Secure the lid and begin heating until steam escapes.

Position the pressure gauge for 15 lb/sq in. and maintain the heat just high enough to cause the gauge to jiggle about 3 times per minute. Continue to cook for 30 minutes. Reduce pressure carefully before removing the gauge and opening the lid.

5. **Pressure saucepan (marinade)**—Using 227 g of marinated beef stew meat, proceed as in 4 above, but use 200 ml of the marinade instead of water for the liquid.

6. **Microwave oven (no marinade)**—Follow the basic formula. Place ingredients in a non-metallic casserole dish; cover and cook for 2 minutes. Then stir the meat, cover, and microwave another 2 minutes. Repeat 2 more times, for a total of 8 minutes of microwave cooking.

7. **Microwave oven (marinade)**—Using ~227 g of the marinated beef stew meat, proceed as in procedure 6, but substitute 200 ml of the marinade for the water.

8. **Dutch oven (no marinade)**—Follow the basic formula. Place in a Dutch oven or heavy pan equipped with tightly fitting lid. Add salt and 200 ml of water. Cover and heat on a range-top unit adjusted to maintain a simmering temperature. Braise until meat is fork tender (approximately 2 to 3 hours).

9. **Dutch oven (marinade)**—Using 227 g of marinated beef, proceed as in procedure 8 above, but substitute 200 ml of marinade for water.

EVALUATION

1. Weigh the meat after cooking, being sure to drain it thoroughly before weighing. Compare the yields. Measure the volume of the drip for each treatment.

2. Subjective evaluation is done by examining the exterior appearance. The beef should have a pleasingly browned, somewhat moist surface. The interior will be a uniform, medium brown. Flavor, juiciness, and tenderness are evaluated by the judges. The number of chews should be counted to aid in assessing tenderness of the samples.

STUDY QUESTIONS

1. Outline the procedure for cooking meat in a slow cooker. What advantages are found for the use of this piece of equipment? What disadvantages?

2. Outline the procedure used for stewing meat in the microwave oven. What advantage(s) are found for the use of this piece of equipment? What disadvantage(s)?

CHART 6.2   MEAT COOKERY—EQUIPMENT VARIATIONS

Treatment	Total cooking loss (%)*	Drip loss (ml)	Appearance	Juiciness	Flavor	Tenderness (# chews)
Slow cooker 1. High heat						
2. Low heat						
3. Low heat, marinade						
Pressure cooker 4. No marinade						
5. Marinade						
Microwave oven 6. No marinade						
7. Marinade						
Dutch oven 8. No marinade						
9. Marinade						

*% total cooking loss = [(original meat wt − cooked meat wt)/(original meat wt)] × 100

Name

ADDITIONAL OBSERVATIONS AND NOTES

3. Outline the procedure for stewing meat in a pressure saucepan. What advantage(s) are found for the use of this piece of equipment? What disadvantages?

4. Are there differences in the yield of meat prepared by the use of the various pieces of equipment? If so, which results in the greatest yield? The lowest yield?

5. Does a wine (acidic) marinade promote tenderness of meats that will be cooked by moist heat? What other possible functions might the marinade perform?

6. Compare the meats cooked by each method for:

   a. Drip loss

   b. Juiciness

   c. Appearance

   d. Flavor

   e. Tenderness

EXPERIMENT 6.3—MEAT TENDERIZERS AND ACID OBJECTIVES

Upon completion of this experiment, you will be able to:

1. Explain the theory of enzymatic tenderizing of connective tissue in meat.
2. Discuss the relative effectiveness of a powdered enzyme (papain), a fresh enzyme (bromelain), and acid (acetic) as tenderizing agents in meat cookery.
3. Evaluate the palatability of meats prepared with the use of tenderizing agents.

BASIC FORMULA—MEAT TENDERIZERS

~110 g (1/14 lb) top round steak

At 1" intervals, cut through the connective tissue surrounding the steak to keep the meat flat during broiling. Weigh the sample and record the weight. (Each sample should be in one piece and need not be exactly the weight suggested.)

It is important to broil all of the meats at the same time. This means that procedures 2, 3, 4, and 5, which require 60 minutes of bench time, should be started first, with the 30 minute samples being started appropriately, and finally the 0 minute samples being prepared. At this point, all samples should be broiled, with groups 1 and 2 together on one broiler pan and the other three groups (3, 4, and 5) each being on a separate broiler pan.

Before preheating the broiler, check the position of the broiler rack to be sure that the upper surface of the meat will be approximately 2" from the heat when the meat is being broiled. Place the meat and broiler pan in the broiler unit, being sure to note and record the time. Broil the first side of the meat 5 minutes. Use tongs to turn the meat, and then broil the second side 3 minutes.

Remove the meat from the broiler, weigh the cut, and then place on a serving dish for evaluation, being sure that the side that was broiled first is on top.

PROCEDURE

1. **Control**—Prepare the basic formula, being sure not to salt the meat. Broil on the same pan with the cuts from procedure 2.

2. **Meat tenderizer**—Prepare 3 pieces of steak according to the basic formula, but use 1 steak for each of the following treatments.

   a. *60 minutes standing*—After weighing the meat, sprinkle 1 g of meat tenderizer over the entire surface of the cut and let stand 1 hour before broiling.

b. *30 minutes standing*—After weighing the meat, sprinkle 1 g meat tenderizer over the surface of the cut and let stand 30 minutes before broiling. (Do this 30 minutes after preparation of 2a.)

c. *0 minutes standing*—After weighing the meat, sprinkle 1 g meat tenderizer over the entire surface of the cut. Place on the broiler pan with the steaks from 2a, 2b, and 1. Broil immediately according to the basic formula.

3. **Meat tenderizer, perforated**—Prepare 3 pieces of steak according to the basic formula, using 1 steak for each of the following treatments.

a. *60 minutes standing*—After weighing the meat, sprinkle 1 g meat tenderizer over the entire surface of the cut. Using a 4-tined table fork, perforate the entire surface deeply 50 times. Allow to stand for 60 minutes.

b. *30 minutes standing*—Prepare meat as in 3a, but time it to stand for only 30 minutes.

c. *0 minutes standing*—Prepare cut as in 3a, but place it on the broiler pan with the cuts from 3a and 3b immediately after perforating 50 times. Broil immediately according to the basic formula.

4. **Acid marinade**—Prepare 3 pieces of round steak according to the basic formula, but use 1 steak for each of the following treatments.

a. *60 minutes standing*—In a small, shallow dish, immerse the steak in undiluted white vinegar for 60 minutes, turning once at the end of 30 minutes. Proceed according to the basic formula.

b. *30 minutes standing*—In a small, shallow dish, immerse the steak in undiluted white vinegar for 30 minutes, turning once at the end of the first 15 minutes. Prepare according to the basic formula.

c. *0 minutes standing*—In a small, shallow dish, immerse the steak in undiluted white vinegar. Immediately turn it over and then place on the broiler pan with 4a and 4b. Proceed according to the basic formula.

5. **Fresh pineapple**—Prepare 3 pieces of steak according to the basic formula, but use 1 steak for each of the following treatments.

a. *60 minutes standing*—In a shallow dish, coat both sides of the steak with pineapple puree prepared from fresh pineapple. Let stand for 30 minutes. Turn the steak after again coating both sides with pineapple puree.

b. *30 minutes standing*—In a shallow dish, coat both sides of the steak with pineapple puree prepared from fresh pineapple. Let stand for 15 minutes. Turn the steak after again coating both sides with pineapple puree, and let stand for another 15 minutes (total marinating time is 30 minutes). Proceed according to the basic formula.

c. *0 minutes standing*—In a shallow dish, coat both sides of the steak with pineapple puree prepared from fresh pineapple. Place on the broiler pan with the cuts from 5a and 5b. Proceed according to the basic formula.

EVALUATION

1. Calculate the cooking losses for each treatment.

2. Exterior evaluation is done before cutting samples. Particular attention should be directed toward noting the texture of the surface. Note also the color and uniformity of color of the surface. Observe the apparent juiciness or dryness of the surface.

3. Interior subjective evaluation includes a comparison of color changes between samples. The texture of the meat and its mouthfeel should be noted. Juiciness and flavor also are evaluated. Tenderness can be judged by counting the number of chews.

STUDY QUESTIONS

1. Explain the theory of enzyme action which is proposed for interpreting the action of enzymes on meats.

2. What substance contained in fresh pineapple is effective in helping to tenderize meats? Could canned pineapple be used in this experiment? Why? Could frozen pineapple be used? Why?

3. Were the two methods of applying the meat tenderizer equally effective in tenderizing steak? Comment on any differences that may have been noted.

4. Compare the efficacy of each of the following in tenderizing steaks. Note also any other differences between treatments that would influence consumer acceptance.

   a. Meat tenderizer sprinkled on the surface

   b. Meat tenderizer perforated into meat

   c. Acid marinade

   d. Fresh pineapple juice on surface

5. Does the time allowed for action of enzymes or acid prior to cooking have any influence on appearance, flavor, juiciness, cooking losses, tenderness, and texture? If so, indicate the influences noted and discuss the possible reasons for these differences.

6. What might be the reason(s) for using the various tenderizing techniques evaluated in this experiment? When might it be wise to use one of the techniques? When might it be better to broil the meat without use of any of these techniques?

CHART 6.3   MEAT TENDERIZERS AND ACID

Treatment	Exterior appearance	Flavor	Juiciness	Texture and mouthfeel	Tenderness (# chews)	Cooking loss (%)*
1. Control						
2. Meat tenderizer a. 60 min.						
b. 30 min.						
c. 0 min.						
3. Meat tenderizer, perforated a. 60 min.						
b. 30 min.						
c. 0 min.						
4. Acid marinade a. 60 min.						
b. 30 min.						
c. 0 min.						
5. Fresh pineapple a. 60 min.						
b. 30 min.						
c. 0 min.						

*% total cooking loss = [(original meat wt − cooked meat wt)/(original meat wt)] × 100

Name

ADDITIONAL OBSERVATIONS AND NOTES

EXPERIMENT 6.4—ROASTING MEAT
OBJECTIVES

Upon completion of the experiment, you will be able to:

1. Compare the advantages and disadvantages of the use of various temperatures for roasting tender cuts of meat.
2. Compare the following palatability factors for roasts cooked with and without aluminum foil (or plastic wrap in microwave oven):
   Appearance
   Flavor
   Juiciness
   Tenderness
3. Describe the impact of use of a coating of rock salt on palatability and cooking losses of beef roasts.
4. Select the preferred roasting method for a tender roast under prescribed conditions, such as limited time for roasting.

BASIC FORMULA–ROAST BEEF

~900 g (2 lb)	Beef roast
	or
454 g (1 lb)	Ground beef (shaped into a loaf)

Weigh the pan and rack; record. Record the total weight of the pan, rack, and meat. Use a skewer to make a hole for the meat thermometer to be inserted. Insert the thermometer so that the bulb is in the center of the roast and turned so that it can be read easily in the oven. Place the pan and roast in the oven with the oven rack adjusted to place the roast close to the middle of the oven. Check to be sure the thermometer can be read easily, preferably without opening the oven door. Roast until the thermometer registers 63°C (145°F). Let the roast stand at room temperature for 5 minutes. Read the thermometer and then remove it. Weigh the roast, pan, rack, and drippings before removing the roast; record. Weigh the pan, rack, and drippings. Calculate the losses (see evaluation chart).

PROCEDURE

1. **200°F (93°C), no foil**—Follow the basic formula. Roast in oven set at 200°F until thermometer reaches 63°C (145°F). Time required will be approximately 8 hours (4 hours for ground beef loaf).

2. **200°F (93°C), foil wrapped**—Follow the basic formula, but first weigh the roast and record the weight. Then wrap the roast in a single layer

of aluminum foil, folding over twice at each seam to make a tight seal. Be sure the thermometer can be read easily. Roast in 200°F oven until thermometer reaches 63°C (145°F). The time required will be about 8 hours for the roast or 4 hours for the ground beef loaf.

3. **325F (163°C), no foil**—Follow the basic formula. Roast in oven at 325°F until the thermometer reaches 63°C (145°F). Time required will be less than 2 hours.

4. **325°F (163°C), foil wrapped**—Follow the basic formula, but first weigh the roast and then wrap in a single layer of aluminum foil, which has been folded over twice at each seam to make a tight seal. Be sure the thermometer can be read easily. Roast in 325°F oven until thermometer reaches 63°C (145°F).

5. **425°F (220°C), no foil**—Follow the basic formula. Roast in oven set at 425°F until thermometer reaches 63°C (145°F). Time reqired will be approximately 1 hour. If possible, this roast should be prepared in a self-cleaning oven.

6. **425°F (220°C), foil wrapped**—Follow the basic formula, but first weigh the roast and then wrap in a single layer of aluminum foil which has been folded over twice at each seam to make a tight seal. Be sure the thermometer can be read easily. Roast at 425°F until the thermometer reaches 63°C (145°F).

7. **Microwave oven, no wrap**—Follow the basic formula. Roast by placing weighed roast in a shallow non-metallic baking dish and leaning the roast against a custard cup if it will not stand upright. Insert special microwave oven thermometer, if available, being sure to put the sensor in the center of the largest muscle. Set timer for 5 minutes. Baste roast when first 5 minutes have elapsed. Turn roast fat side up, cover with wax paper, and set timer for 5 1/2 minutes. If possible, monitor the temperature rise during this period. Remove the roast when the temperature indicates 130°F (55°C). Let the roast stand for 20 minutes with the wax paper still covering it. Note the temperature at 5-minute intervals throughout the 20-minute period.

8. **Microwave oven, plastic wrap**—Wrap the roast in plastic wrap. Cut a slit 1" long in the upper portion of the wrapping to permit some loss of steam. Be sure the thermometer is inserted carefully. Cook according to the direction in procedure 7. It is not necessary to place wax paper over the roast during the second roasting period.

9. **Rock salt coating, 325°F (163°C)**—Follow the basic formula, but weigh the roast initially and again after coating it heavily with rock salt. Following roasting, complete the basic formula weighings and then knock off all of the salt before finally weighing the roast.

10. **Rock salt coating, 500°F (260°C) for 15 minutes, then 325°F (163°C)**—Follow directions for Procedure 9, but roast for 15 minutes at 500°F (260°C) and then reduce temperature to 325°F (163°C) for remainder of the roasting period.

EVALUATION

1. Calculate the total cooking loss, the % loss, and the drip loss for each method.

2. Note the roasting time required for each roast.

3. Exterior evaluation is based on color, uniformity of color, retention of shape, and moistness of surface.

4. Palatability is based on juiciness, flavor, color, and tenderness. Tenderness can be evaluated by counting the number of chews. Color evaluation can encompass the uniformity of color from the exterior to the interior, as well as the actual color.

STUDY QUESTIONS

1. Which temperature resulted in the greatest losses during roasting? What effect, if any, does aluminum foil have on cooking losses?

2. Does the use of aluminum foil have a uniform effect on retarding the rate of cooking at all of the oven temperatures tested?

3. Was the temperature rise after the roast was taken from the oven uniform for all treatments? If not, analyze the differences and predict what the temperature rise after roasting would be in an oven set at 232°C (450°F).

4. Compare roasts prepared with and without foil at the same oven temperatures for:

   a. Exterior appearance

   b. Flavor

   c. Juiciness

   d. Interior color

   e. Tenderness

5. Compare the unwrapped roasts prepared at the 3 oven settings and in the microwave oven for:

   a. Exterior appearance

   b. Flavor

   c. Juiciness

   d. Interior color

   e. Tenderness

6. Compare the wrapped roasts prepared at the 3 oven settings and in the microwave oven for:

   a. Exterior appearance

   b. Flavor

   c. Juiciness

   d. Interior color

   e. Tenderness

Chart 6.4.1   Beef Roasts—Cooking Losses and Roasting Times

Treatment	Weight pan + rack (g)	Cooking time	Weight pan + rack + drip. (g)	Final interior temp.	Cooking losses				
					Meat weight		Total[3] loss (g)	Total[4] (%)	Drip-pings[5,6] (g and %)
					Raw[1] (g)	Cooked[2] (g)			
200°F (93°C) 1. No foil									
2. Foil									
325°F (163°C) 3. No foil									
4. Foil									
425°F (220°C) 5. No foil									
6. Foil									
Microwave oven 7. No wrap									
8. Plastic wrap									
Rock salt 9. 325°F (163°C)									
10. 500°F (260°C) 15 min; then 325°F (163°C)									

[1] Raw weight = (weight pan + racks + meat) − (weight pan + racks)
[2] Cooked weight = (weight pan + rack + cooked meat + drippings) − (weight pan + rack + drippings)
[3] Total cooking loss = raw weight − cooked weight
[4] % loss = (total cooking loss/raw weight) × 100
[5] Drippings = (weight pan + rack + drippings) − (weight pan + rack)
[6] % drippings = (drippings/raw weight) × 100

Name

ADDITIONAL OBSERVATIONS AND NOTES

CHART 6.4.2   BEEF ROASTS–PALATABILITY

Treatment	Exterior appearance	Retention of shape	Flavor	Juiciness	Interior color	Tenderness (# chews)
200°F (93°C) 1. No foil						
2. Foil						
325°F (163°C) 3. No foil						
4. Foil						
425°F (220°C) 5. No foil						
6. Foil						
Microwave oven 7. No wrap						
8. Plastic wrap						
Rock Salt 9. 325°F (163°C)						

10. 500°F (260°C)
   15 min; then
   325°F (163°C)						

Name

ADDITIONAL OBSERVATIONS AND NOTES

EXPERIMENT 6.5—BAKED FISH OR CHICKEN
OBJECTIVES

Upon completion of the experiment, you will be able to:

1. Discuss the relationship between baking temperatures and palatability of fish and chicken dishes.
2. Trace the change in palatability that occur as fish steaks and chicken are heated to higher interior temperatures.
3. Compare fish and chicken baked in microwave ovens and in conventional ovens; comparisons to include time required, palatability, and methods recommended.

BASIC FORMULA–BAKED FISH OR CHICKEN

1 Fish steak (1″ thick) or 1/2 Chicken breast

Record the weight of the rack and pan before placing fish or chicken on rack. Record the weight of the rack, pan, and meat. Insert thermometer so it can be read easily during baking. Place the pan with its rack and meat on the rack in the center of the oven. Bake at assigned temperature until meat thermometer reaches 75°C (167°F) unless otherwise indicated in the assigned procedure. Record the weight of the baked meat, pan, rack, and drippings; then weigh the pan, rack, and drippings without the meat.

PROCEDURE

1. **300°F (149°C), no foil**—Follow the basic formula, baking at 300°F (149°C). Note the time required to reach the interior temperature of 75°C.

2. **300°F (149°C), foil wrapped**—Follow the basic formula, except wrap the weighed fish or chicken in a single layer of aluminum foil, being careful to fold the seams 2 times to make a tight seal. Bake at 300°F. Note the time required to reach the interior temperature of 75°C.

3. **350°F (177°C), no foil**—Follow the basic formula, baking at 350°F (177°C). Note the time required to reach the interior temperature of 75°C.

4. **350°F (177°C), foil wrapped**—Follow the basic formula, except wrap the weighed fish or chicken in a single layer of aluminum foil, being careful to fold any seams 2 times to make a tight seal. Bake at 400°F. Note the time required to reach the interior temperature of 75°C.

5. **400°F (204°C), no foil**—Follow the basic formula, baking in an oven set at 400°F (204°C). Note the time required to reach the interior temperature of 75°C.

6. **400°F (204°C), foil wrapped**—Follow the basic formula, except wrap the weighed fish or chicken in a single layer of aluminum foil, being careful to fold any seams 2 times to make a tight seal. Bake at 400°F. Note the time required to reach the interior temperature of 75°C.

7. **Microwave oven, no wrap**—Weigh the fish or chicken. Place in a non-metallic dish. Be sure to position the microwave oven thermometer so that it can be read while the meat is baking. If this is not possible, the oven should be set for periods of 1 minute and the temperature checked so that cooking can be stopped at a temperature of 73°C (to allow for a small temperature rise to 75°C after baking is completed). If a thermometer is not available, microwave the fish for a total time of 3 1/2 minutes and use a laboratory thermometer to determine the interior temperature.

8. **Microwave oven, plastic wrap**—Follow procedure 7, except wrap fish or chicken in a layer of plastic wrap and cut a slit 1″ long in the wrap.

9. **70°C interior temperature**—Follow the basic formula, baking at 350°F (without foil) until the interior temperature is 70°C;

10. **80°C interior temperature**—Follow the basic formula, baking at 350°F (without foil) until the interior temperature is 80°C.

11. **85°C interior temperature**—Follow the basic formula, baking at 350°F (no foil) until the interior temperature is 85°C.

EVALUATION

1. Compare the cooking losses for the various treatments.

2. *Exterior evaluation* includes the appearance of the surface and any exudates from the flesh.

3. *Interior evaluation* includes subjective evaluation of texture, tenderness, and juiciness of the flesh. Ideally, fish should be moist, very tender, and the flesh should flake when manipulated with a fork. Tenderness can be evaluated by counting the number of chews. Juiciness can be determined subjectively by judges or objectively by the use of a pressometer or hydraulic press, if either is available. Drip loss provides another approach to determining juiciness.

STUDY QUESTIONS

1. What cookery method produces the most palatable baked fish or chicken? Why?

2. Describe the effect(s) of aluminum foil on the preparation and palatability of baked fish or chicken.

CHART 6.5 BAKED FISH OR CHICKEN—VARIATIONS IN BAKING AND INTERIOR TEMPERATURES

Treatment	Cooking loss[1] (%)	Drip loss[2] (g)	Time (min)	Appearance		Texture	Tenderness (# chews)	Juiciness
				Surface	Exudate			
300°F 1. No foil								
2. Foil								
350°F 3. No foil								
4. Foil								
400°F 5. No foil								
6. Foil								
Microwave oven 7. No wrap								
8. Plastic wrap								
350°F oven, no foil 9. 70°C interior								
10. 80°C interior								
11. 85°C interior								

[1] Cooking loss (%) = {[(wt. pan + rack + fish) − (wt. pan + rack + cooked fish)]/[(wt. pan + rack + fish) − (wt. pan + rack)]} × 100

[2] % drip loss = [(wt. pan + rack + drippings) − (wt. pan + rack)]/(raw wt.) × 100

ADDITIONAL OBSERVATIONS AND NOTES

3. What changes can be detected as the interior temperature of baked fish is increased? Theorize regarding the causes of the changes.

4. How do the baking losses noted in baking fish or chicken compare with those found in the experiment on baking beef? What explanation can be postulated for the difference(s)?

5. Compare the results of the better microwave method with those from the preferred method of baking fish in a conventional oven. What advantages and disadvantages are evident for each type of cookery?

6. Compare the results obtained in the fish and chicken experiments if both were tested.

EXPERIMENT 6.6—TOFU
OBJECTIVES

Upon completion of the experiment, you will be able to:

1. Identify various forms of tofu and describe their characteristics.
2. Explain the procedures that need to be followed to maintain the safety and quality of tofu.
3. Discuss the suitability of various types of tofu in making dips, pie fillings, stir-fry recipes, and soups.

PROCEDURE

Safety and care of fresh tofu   Tofu is perishable (unless it is packaged aseptically) and must be kept refrigerated. The expiration date needs to be heeded. Opened packages of tofu require care: (1) rinsing and then covering with fresh water daily, and (2) storing in the refrigerator no more than 1 week. Frozen tofu can be stored up to 6 months.

Pressing   If tofu needs to hold its shape in a product, it should be pressed to remove excess water before being added to other ingredients. To press tofu, remove it from its water-filled storage container and place in a pie plate. Top the block of tofu with another plate and add heavy cans to the plate to apply pressure on the tofu for at least 15 minutes. Pour off the expressed water before removing the tofu.

BASIC FORMULA—ONION DIP

100 g	Tofu
2 g	Dry onion soup mix

Place ingredients in blender and whirl just until the tofu is smooth.

PROCEDURE

1. **Tofu dips**

   a. *Soft silken tofu*—Prepare the basic formula using soft silken tofu.

   b. *Regular tofu*—Prepare the basic formula using regular tofu. If the dip is too stiff, measure and record the amount of water added to achieve a dip consistency.

   c. *Firm silken tofu*—Prepare the basic formula using firm silken tofu. If the dip is too stiff, measure and record the amount of water added to achieve a dip consistency.

d. *Miso*—Prepare the basic formula using miso for the tofu. If the dip is too stiff, measure and record the amount of water added to achieve a dip consistency.

BASIC FORMULA—CHOCOLATE PIE FILLING

225 g	Chocolate chips
40 ml	Light corn syrup
225 g	Firm silken tofu
225 g	Soft silken tofu

Carefully melt chocolate chips before stirring in corn syrup. Meanwhile puree tofus until smooth. Stir in chip mixture. Pour into custard cups and refrigerate until evaluated.

---

2. **Tofu pie filling**

   a. *Firm and soft silken tofu (control)*—Prepare the basic formula.

   b. *Firm silken tofu*—Prepare the basic formula, but use 450 g firm silken tofu and 0 g soft silken tofu.

   c. *Soft silken tofu*—Prepare the basic formula, but use 0 g firm silken tofu and 450 g soft silken tofu.

BASIC FORMULA—STIR-FRY TOFU

15 ml	Olive oil
50 g	Celery (cut in matchsticks 1″ long)
20 g	Green onion, thinly sliced
160 g	Tomato, chopped
90 g	Zucchini, thinly sliced
150 g	Firm tofu, 1/2″ cubes
20 ml	Soy sauce

Heat frying pan and olive oil 30 seconds. Add all vegetables and tofu; fry over moderate heat with gentle stirring for 4 minutes. Add soy sauce and stir for 20 seconds before serving.

---

3. **Stir-fry tofu**

   a. *Firm tofu (control)*—Prepare the basic formula.

   b. *Regular tofu*—Prepare the basic formula, but use regular tofu.

   c. *Soft tofu*—Prepare the basic formula, but use soft tofu.

BASIC FORMULA—GREEN ONION AND TOFU SOUP

450 ml	Water
7.4 g	Chicken bouillon cube
20 g	Green onion, thinly sliced
150 g	Firm tofu, 1/2" cubes

Heat water and bouillon cube to boiling. Add onion and tofu; simmer 50 seconds. Serve.

---

4. **Soup with tofu**

a. *Firm tofu (control)*—Prepare basic formula.

b. *Regular tofu*—Prepare basic formula, but use regular tofu.

EVALUATION

Subjectively evaluate all of the products, noting specific characteristics that distinguish each of the samples from their counterparts (e.g., the four samples of dip). Concentrate particularly upon textural qualities and describe each product with words that accurately depict the mouthfeel. Note flavor impressions.

STUDY QUESTIONS

1. What is tofu? Miso? What organoleptic characteristic(s) enabled you to distinguish between tofu and miso in dip products in this experiment?

2. What are the advantages/disadvantages of making a dip using (a) soft tofu, (b) regular tofu, (c) firm silken tofu, and (d) miso?

3. Which of the tofu variations did you prefer for making the pie filling? Why? Would you recommend this filling? Explain your answer.

4. Describe the qualities tofu adds to a stir-fry dish. Which type of tofu was best suited to this application?

5. Describe the tofu cubes in the soup. Which cubes did you prefer? Why?

6. Identify suitable applications for these types of tofus: (a) soft, (b) regular, (c) firm, (d) soft silken, and (e) firm silken.

CHART 6.6 TOFU

Tofu	Aroma	Flavor	Textural qualities	Palatability
1. Dips a. Soft silken				
b. Regular				
c. Firm silken				
d. Miso				
2. Pie filling a. Firm and soft silken				
b. Firm silken				
c. Soft silken				
3. Stir-fry a. Firm				
b. Regular				
c. Soft				
4. Soup a. Firm				
b. Regular				

Name

ADDITIONAL OBSERVATIONS AND NOTES

7
Eggs

Eggs serve a variety of purposes in food preparation. Uses include individual egg dishes prepared either in or out of the shell (hard and soft cooked eggs, poached, baked, and scrambled), omelets, and creamed eggs. In addition, eggs are utilized as (a) thickening agents in hollandaise and other sauces, (b) emulsifying agents in mayonnaise and other recipes, and (c) foams in angel and sponge cakes, soufflés, and other foam products.

Eggs contribute flavor to products. When the yolk is used, the color also is changed. The texture of egg-containing foods will be modified when the yolk emulsifies other ingredients, when the proteins are denatured, and when foams are utilized. These contributions will be influenced by the quality of the eggs that are used.

Fresh eggs commonly are used to prepare recipes, but other forms of eggs also are available. Egg substitutes are used by many people seeking ways to reduce dietary cholesterol. Other forms of eggs that may be used in food preparation include dried eggs (whole, yolks, or whites) and frozen eggs (whole, yolks, or whites). The experiments in this chapter include use of some of these forms of eggs to illustrate the cooking characteristics of these alternatives.

EXPERIMENT 7.1—EGGS IN THE SHELL
OBJECTIVES

Upon completion of the experiment, you will be able to:

1. Identify changes occurring in eggs as they deteriorate.
2. Outline the preferred method for cooking eggs in the shell.
3. Explain the relationship of time and temperature in the denaturation of egg proteins.
4. Minimize the likelihood of forming a ferrous sulfide ring in hard cooked eggs.

BASIC FORMULA—HARD COOKED EGGS

2 c	Water
2	Eggs

Heat 2 c water to the temperature required. Then use a slotted spoon to add 2 eggs. Continue to heat at the assigned temperature for the designated length of time. Cool one egg at room temperature. Cool the other egg under a stream of cold running water for 3 minutes. Fill the pan with cold water and let egg cool in the pan, changing the water whenever it seems warm.

PROCEDURE

1. **Fresh, 85°C, 30 min.**—Following the basic formula, prepare 2 eggs at 85°C for 30 minutes.

2. **Fresh, 95°C, 20 min.**—Following the basic formula, simmer 2 eggs at 95°C 20 minutes.

3. **Deteriorated, 95°C, 20 min.**—Using 2 deteriorated eggs, follow the basic formula; simmer at 95°C for 20 minutes.

4. **Fresh, boiling, 13 min.**—Following the basic formula, boil 2 eggs for 13 minutes.

5. **Deteriorated, boiling, 13 min.**—Using 2 deteriorated eggs, follow the basic formula; boil for 13 minutes.

6. **Pressure saucepan, 5 min.**—Place 2 fresh eggs and 2 deteriorated eggs (shells marked with a D to identify the deteriorated eggs) in a pressure saucepan containing 1 c water. Secure the cover according to directions, position the pressure gauge for 15 pounds, and heat to that pressure. Heat to maintain 15 pounds pressure (follow pressure saucepan directions) for 5 minutes. Hold the pressure saucepan under cold running water to reduce the pressure (again following directions for pressure saucepan being used). When pressure is reduced, remove the gauge and the lid. Cool 1 fresh and 1 deteriorated egg under cold running water; cool the remaining 2 eggs at room temperature.

EVALUATION

1. Carefully peel the eggs and cut in half lengthwise.

2. Place halves on labeled plates. Remove the yolk of one half and place the cut side down so the curved outer portion is upward.

3. Note the color of the curved side of the yolk.

4. Compare the location of the yolk within the white of the deteriorated egg with that of the comparable fresh egg.

CHART 7.1 EGGS COOKED IN THE SHELL

Treatment	Fast cool		Room temperature cool	
	Yolk	White	Yolk	White
1. Fresh, 85°C, 30 min.				
2. Fresh, 95°C, 20 min.				
3. Deteriorated, 95°C, 20 min.				
4. Fresh, boiling, 13 min.				
5. Deteriorated, boiling, 13 min.				
6. a. Fresh, 15 lb pressure, 121°C, 5 min.				
6. b. Deteriorated, 15 lb pressure, 121°C, 5 min.				

Name

ADDITIONAL OBSERVATIONS AND NOTES

5. Compare the size of the air space of the deteriorated egg with that of the fresh egg.

6. Use very small samples of the yolk and white to compare the flavors of the deteriorated with the fresh eggs.

STUDY QUESTIONS

1. Which treatment resulted in the least formation of ferrous sulfide around the yolk? Why?

2. Describe the differences that can be observed between fresh and deteriorated eggs (include flavor changes).

3. Why were the eggs cooked in the pressure saucepan cooked a shorter time than those in boiling water? What changes would you expect to find in an egg cooked in a pressure saucepan for 13 minutes at 15 pounds pressure?

4. Outline the method you consider to be the best way to hard cook eggs. State the reasons for this choice.

EXPERIMENT 7.2—EGGS OUT OF THE SHELL
OBJECTIVES

Upon completion of the experiment, you will be able to:

1. Explain the effect of salt in the water used for poaching eggs.
2. Explain the effect of vinegar in water used for poaching eggs.
3. Identify the advantages of using fresh eggs for poaching.
4. Compare the palatability of scrambled eggs made with fresh eggs, deteriorated eggs, and egg substitutes.
5. Interpret the effect of dilution of egg protein in the preparation of scrambled eggs.
6. Discuss the desirability of various rates of heating eggs during scrambling.
7. Evaluate poached and scrambled eggs and outline the preferred method for preparing each.

BASIC FORMULA—POACHED EGGS

2 c	Water
1	Egg

Bring 2 c water to a boil in a 1-qt saucepan. Break 1 egg into a saucer, quickly note characteristics, and slide it gently from the saucer into the water. Maintain a high simmer for 3 minutes, but do not boil. Immediately remove the egg, using a slotted spoon.

PROCEDURE

1. **Poached eggs**

   a. *Fresh egg*—Follow basic formula.

   b. *Deteriorated egg*—Follow the basic formula, but use a deteriorated egg.

   c. *Salt in water*—Follow the basic formula, but add 3/4 tsp salt to the cooking water.

   d. *Deteriorated, salt in water*—Follow the basic formula using a deteriorated egg, but add 3/4 tsp salt to the cooking water.

   e. *Acid in water*—Follow the basic formula, but add 1 tsp vinegar to the cooking water.

   f. *Deteriorated, acid in water*—Follow the basic formula using a deteriorated egg, but add 1 tsp vinegar to the cooking water.

   g. *Acid and salt*—Follow the basic formula, but add 3/4 tsp salt and 1 tsp vinegar to cooking water.

   h. *Deteriorated, acid and salt*—Follow the basic formula using a deteriorated egg, but add 3/4 tsp salt and 1 tsp vinegar to the cooking water.

i. *Swirl water*—Follow the basic formula, but swirl the boiling water around the pan to create a vortex before sliding the egg into the water.

j. *Deteriorated, swirl water*—Follow the basic formula using a deteriorated egg, but swirl the water around the pan to create a vortex before sliding the egg into the water.

BASIC FORMULA—SCRAMBLED EGGS

48 g (1)	Egg
15 ml (1 tbsp)	Milk
dash (1/16 tsp)	Salt
9 g (1 tsp)	Margarine

Gently beat together egg, milk, and salt. Melt margarine in very small frying pan on thermostatic unit set at 200°F. Heat until the pan is hot, but the fat is not smoking. Add egg mixture. Continue cooking at 200°F, stirring slowly to scrape egg in large pieces from bottom and sides of pan. Note the cooking time required. Transfer to a funnel (supported by a ring stand) lined with filter paper positioned above a graduated cylinder. Drain eggs in funnel for 10 minutes. Place eggs on plate for evaluation. Record the amount of syneresis.

---

2. **Scrambled eggs**

a. *Control*—Prepare scrambled egg as stated in the basic formula.

b. *Higher temperature*—Prepare the basic formula, but cook at 325°F.

c. *Fast stir*—Prepare the basic formula, but stir rapidly.

d. *Double boiler*—Prepare the basic formula, but cook in a double boiler, as follows. Bring 2 cups of water to a boil in the *bottom* of a double boiler while melting the margarine in the *upper part.* When water is boiling and the margarine is melted, add the egg mixture to the upper part. Cook over boiling water while stirring slowly until egg is coagulated but still shiny.

e. *No milk*—Prepare the basic formula, but omit milk.

f. *Extra milk*—Prepare the basic formula, but use 30 ml milk.

g. *Deteriorated egg*—Prepare the basic formula, but use deteriorated egg.

h. *Egg substitute*—Prepare the basic formula, but use 48 g of an egg substitute in place of the fresh egg. (Repeat for each egg substitute.)

i. *Omega-3*—Prepare the basic formula using omega-3 eggs.

EVALUATION

Poached eggs are evaluated on the basis of their appearance (white holding together well and piling around and over yolk), the white being completely coagulated, yet tender, and the yolk slightly thickened. In addition, the flavor should be fresh and pleasing.

Scrambled eggs should be a homogeneous yellow color throughout, with no traces of white and no areas of brown on the surface. The pieces should be rather large, tender, and slightly moist on the surface, but with no liquid separating from them.

STUDY QUESTIONS

1. Does the addition of salt to the water used for poaching eggs influence the egg in any way? If so, how? Why does it have this effect?

2. Is it beneficial to add vinegar to the water used in poaching eggs? What causes this effect? What other acids might be used?

3. Are deteriorated eggs satisfactory for poaching? Why or why not?

4. Are deteriorated eggs satisfactory for scrambling? Why or why not?

5. Are (a) egg substitutes and (b) omega-3 eggs satisfactory for scrambling? Explain your answer.

6. What change(s) can be observed when the level of milk used in scrambled eggs is varied from no milk to the equivalent of 2 tbsp per egg?

7. What changes, if any, can be noted at the various temperatures used in scrambling eggs in this experiment? What condition is judged to give the best result?

8. Describe the best method for preparing poached eggs; for preparing scrambled eggs.

CHART 7.2 POACHED EGGS

Treatment	Appearance of yolk	Consistency of white	Tenderness	Flavor
a. Fresh (control)				
b. Deteriorated				
Salt in water c. Fresh				
d. Deteriorated				
Acid in water e. Fresh				
f. Deteriorated				
Acid and salt g. Fresh				
h. Deteriorated				
Swirling water i. Fresh				
j. Deteriorated				

Name

ADDITIONAL OBSERVATIONS AND NOTES

CHART 7.3 SCRAMBLED EGGS

Treatment	Cooking time	Syneresis (ml)	Appearance	Tenderness
a. 200°F (control)				
b. 325°F				
c. Fast stir				
d. Double boiler				
e. No milk				
f. 2x milk				
g. Deteriorated egg				
h. Substitute, type: _____				
i. Omega-3				

Name

ADDITIONAL OBSERVATIONS AND NOTES

EXPERIMENT 7.3—CUSTARDS
OBJECTIVES

Upon completion of the experiment, you will be able to:

1. Interpret the interrelationship between rate of heating and the coagulation temperature of egg proteins.
2. Identify differences in the characteristics of egg white and yolk proteins.
3. Interpret the role of acid in the coagulation of egg proteins.
4. Interpret the role of salts in the coagulation of egg proteins.
5. Interpret the role of sugar in modifying coagulation of egg proteins.
6. Interpret the effect of the concentration of protein on the coagulation temperature of egg proteins.
7. Describe the preferred method for preparing stirred and baked custards.
8. Evaluate stirred and baked custards.

BASIC FORMULA—CUSTARDS

	Stirred custard	*Baked custard*
	237 ml (1c) Milk	355 ml (1 1/2 c) Milk
	48 g (1) Egg	72 g (1 1/2) Egg
	25 g (2 tbsp) Sugar	38 g (3 tbsp) Sugar
	dash (1/16 tsp) Salt	dash (1/12 tsp) Salt

Combine the ingredients by beating gently with an egg beater just enough to blend. Strain to remove chalazae.

Stirred Custard
Pour custard mixture into top of a double boiler. Place above the bottom section, which contains 1 1/2″ water heated to 95°C. Note the time. Heat, stirring continuously with a wooden spoon. Maintain the water in the bottom of the double boiler at a high simmer. Remove a 2 tbsp-sample when the custard is heated to 80°C, 84°C, 88°C, and when it curdles. Use a soup ladle to transfer the samples into glasses clearly labeled with the temperature and the cooking time. Record the cooking time for each temperature, and report the time and temperature when the custard curdled.

Baked Custard
Preheat oven to 177°C (350°F). Divide the custard equally into 3 custard cups, arrange cups in cake pan, and place in oven. Pour boiling water in cake pan to the level of the custards. Insert a laboratory thermometer in one of the custards (supporting it with an oven rack placed in the next position above the custards). Be sure the thermometer can be read easily, preferably without opening the oven door. Record the time and temperature of the custard at the beginning of baking and again every 10 minutes throughout the baking period. Remove 1 custard when the temperature is 80°C, 1 at 84°C, and the last at 88°C.

PROCEDURE

Stirred Custards

1. **Control**—Prepare the basic formula for stirred custard; follow the directions outlined.

2. **Faster cooking rate**—Prepare the basic formula for stirred custard except place the custard over *boiling* water and be sure to maintain an active boil during the entire experiment. Follow the directions outlined for stirred custards.

3. **Yolks**—Prepare basic formula for stirred custard except use 48 g of egg yolk in place of the whole egg. Follow the directions for stirred custards.

4. **Whites**—Prepare the basic formula for stirred custard except use 48 g of egg white in place of the whole egg. Follow the directions outlined for stirred custard.

5. **Increased egg**—Prepare the basic formula for stirred custard except use 96 g of whole egg (instead of 48 g). Follow the directions outlined for stirred custard.

6. **Egg substitute**—Prepare the basic formula for stirred custard, except use 48 g of an egg substitute in place of the whole egg. Follow the directions outlined for stirred custard.

Baked Custards

1. **Control**—Prepare the basic formula for baked custard. Plot the time-temperature data in Chart 7.3.3 (p. 183), using a square as the symbol to record each data point.

2. **No sugar**—Prepare the basic formula for baked custard, but omit sugar.

3. **Double sugar**—Prepare the basic formula for baked custard, but use a total of 76 g of sugar.

4. **Double egg**—Prepare the basic formula for baked custard, but use a total of 144 g of whole egg.

5. **Yolk**—Prepare the basic formula for baked custard, but substitute 72 g of egg yolk in place of the whole egg.

6. **Whites**—Prepare the basic formula for baked custard, but substitute 72 g of whites in place of the whole egg.

7. **Distilled water**—Prepare the basic formula for baked custard, but substitute distilled water (355 ml) in place of milk and omit salt.

8. **Calcium chloride**—Prepare the basic formula for baked custard, but substitute distilled water (355 ml) in place of milk and omit salt. After removing from oven, add 0.3 g calcium chloride to each custard. Stir in until dissolved. Let stand at least 1 minute before evaluating.

9. **Egg substitute**—Prepare the basic formula for baked custard, but use 72 g egg substitute in place of the egg.

10. **Frozen egg whites**—Prepare the basic formula for baked custard, but use 72 g thawed frozen egg whites in place of the whole egg.

11. **Frozen egg yolks**—Prepare the basic formula for baked custard, but use 72 g thawed frozen egg yolks and omit the salt.

12. **Acid**—Prepare the basic formula for baked custard, but use 8 ml lemon juice and 347 ml milk.

13. **Bake at 150°C**—Prepare the basic formula for baked custard, but bake at 300°F (150°C). Plot data on Chart 7.3.3 (p. 183), using a circle to record each data point.

14. **Bake at 232°C**—Prepare the basic formula for baked custard, but bake at 450°F (232°C). Plot data on Chart 7.3.3 (p. 183), using a triangle to record each data point.

EVALUATION

1. *Stirred custards* are evaluated on the basis of color, flavor, and consistency. Perform the line-spread test (see Appendix D) on the most viscous sample from each variable to measure viscosity. This is done by arranging a flat piece of glass on a paper marked with concentric circles, the smallest of which is 2″ in diameter, with each circle 1/8″ larger. A metal ring 2″ in diameter is positioned in the center of the circles and filled to the top with the stirred custard. The ring then is lifted and the custard is allowed to flow for exactly 2 minutes before the flow distance is measured at 4 points (every 90°). The 4 values are averaged to determine the viscosity of the sample. The smaller the value, the more viscous the sample.

2. *Baked custards* are evaluated on color, flavor, syneresis, and tenderness. Subjective evaluations for these characteristics can be made. Objective tests also are useful. Tenderness can be evaluated objectively by use of the penetrometer or by determining percent sag.

   Penetrometer readings are done by chilling the custards a uniform length of time (an hour in the refrigerator is suggested) before testing. The surface skin is taken off before using the penetrometer. Test conditions need to be decided when the first product is tested, and then these conditions need to be used for testing the other samples so that they can all be compared. For example, place a 35-g cone barely touching the surface of the custard (with the penetrometer gauge correctly positioned at 0) and then release the cone for 5 seconds to determine the reading. Tenderness of different samples can be compared if they are tested under identical circumstances. The larger the reading, the more tender the custard gel.

   Percent sag is determined by measuring the heights of the molded and unmolded custards. The calculation is:

$$\% \text{ sag} = \frac{\text{molded height} - \text{unmolded height}}{\text{molded height}} \times 100$$

The larger the percent sag, the more tender the gel.

Syneresis can be measured by placing 1/4 of each of the custards (after testing for tenderness) on individual wire screens placed on empty cups. Collect the liquid and measure the volume of each after 1 hour.

STUDY QUESTIONS

1. Discuss the effect of each of the following upon coagulation temperature of egg mixtures: (a) rate of heating, (b) type and amount of egg protein, (c) acid, (d) salts, (e) freezing of yolks or whites, (f) amount of sugar, and (g) quality of egg.

2. Explain the role of salts in the coagulation of egg mixtures.

3. Explain the role of acid in the coagulation of egg mixtures.

4. Would it be necessary to add more acid to a deteriorated egg than to a fresh egg to achieve the same pH? Why?

5. What method and ratio of ingredients would result in the best stirred custard? In the best baked custard? Explain the reasons for selecting each.

6. Compare the tenderness of each variable used in preparing baked custards with the tenderness of the control baked custard.

7. Compare the color, flavor, and tenderness of baked custards made from whole eggs with those made using: (a) yolks only, (b) whites only, and (c) egg substitutes.

8. Describe and explain the influence, if any, on baked custards if the following types of egg are used: (a) frozen yolks, (b) frozen whites.

9. Which final baking temperature is best for each treatment used in the baked custard experiment?

10. Compare the syneresis from the control baked custard with each of the variables tested in the baked custard sequence. Which treatment had the least syneresis? Which had the most syneresis?

11. Describe a high quality stirred custard. How might such a product be used?

CHART 7.3.1 STIRRED CUSTARDS

Treatment	Temperature (min.)	Color and consistency	Flavor	Line-spread
1. Control* a. 80°C				
b. 84°C			XXX	
c. 88°C			XXX	
d. Curd, _____°C			XXX	
2. Boiling water a. 80°C				
b. 84°C			XXX	
c. 88°C			XXX	
d. Curd, _____°C			XXX	
3. Yolks only a. 80°C				
b. 84°C			XXX	
c. 88°C			XXX	
d. Curd, _____°C			XXX	
4. Whites only a. 80°C				
b. 84°C			XXX	
c. 88°C			XXX	
d. Curd, _____°C			XXX	
5. Extra egg a. 80°C				
b. 84°C			XXX	
c. 88°C			XXX	
d. Curd, _____°C			XXX	
6. Egg substitute a. 80°C				
b. 84°C			XXX	
c. 88°C			XXX	
d. Curd, _____°C			XXX	

* Control

Name

ADDITIONAL OBSERVATIONS AND NOTES

CHART 7.3.2 BAKED CUSTARDS

Treatment	Penetrometer (or % sag)	Syneresis (ml)	Surface	Color and consistency	Flavor
1. Control 177°C a. 80°C					
b. 84°C					XXX
c. 88°C					XXX
2. No sugar a. 80°C					
b. 84°C					XXX
c. 88°C					XXX
3. 2x sugar a. 80°C					
b. 84°C					XXX
c. 88°C					XXX
4. 2x egg a. 80°C					
b. 84°C					XXX
c. 88°C					XXX
5. Yolks a. 80°C					
b. 84°C					XXX
c. 88°C					XXX
6. Whites a. 80°C					
b. 84°C					XXX
c. 88°C					XXX
7. Distilled water (no salt) a. 80°C	XXX	XXX			
b. 84°C	XXX	XXX			XXX
c. 88°C		XXX			XXX
8. CaCl$_2$ a. 80°C					XXX
b. 84°C					XXX
c. 88°C					XXX

Name

ADDITIONAL OBSERVATIONS AND NOTES

CHART 7.3.2 BAKED CUSTARDS (CONTINUED)

Treatment	Penetrometer (or % sag)	Syneresis (ml)	Surface	Color and consistency	Flavor
9. Egg substitute a. 80°C					
b. 84°C					XXX
c. 88°C					XXX
10. Frozen white a. 80°C					
b. 84°C					XXX
c. 88°C					XXX
11. Frozen yolks a. 80°C					
b. 84°C					XXX
c. 88°C					XXX
12. Acid a. 80°C					
b. 84°C					XXX
c. 88°C					XXX
13. 150°C a. 80°C					
b. 84°C					XXX
c. 88°C					XXX
14. 232°C a. 80°C					
b. 84°C					XXX
c. 88°C					XXX

Name

ADDITIONAL OBSERVATIONS AND NOTES

CHART 7.3.3 BAKED CUSTARDS — GRAPH OF TEMPERATURE VERSUS TIME

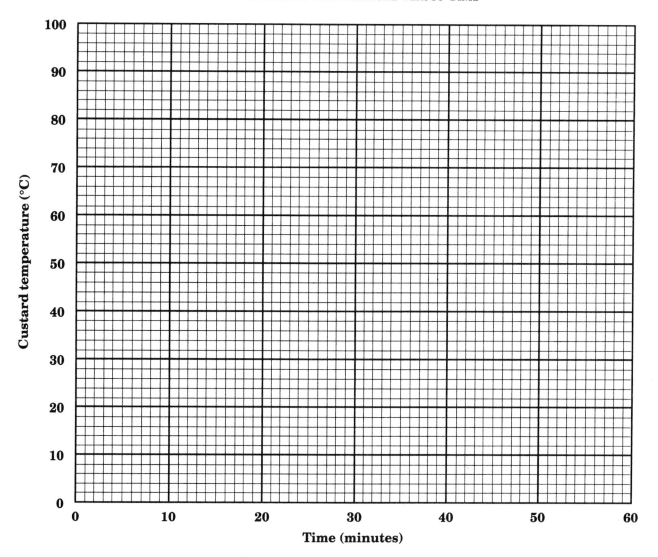

Custard temperature (°C) vs. Time (minutes)

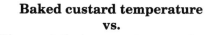

Baked custard temperature
vs.
Times at three oven temperatures
O _____ 150°C
▢ - - - - 177°C
Δ . . . . . 232°C

ADDITIONAL OBSERVATIONS AND NOTES

12. Describe a high quality baked custard. Suggest some variations for serving baked custards.

13. Compare the times required for the custards to reach 84°C when baked in an oven at (a) 150°C, (b) 177°C, (c) 232°C. Explain why custards are more likely to be overbaked when the oven temperature is at 232°C than at 177°C (see Chart 7.3.3).

EXPERIMENT 7.4—HOLLANDAISE SAUCE
OBJECTIVES

Upon completion of the experiment, you will be able to:

1. Explain the roles of egg yolk in the preparation of hollandaise sauce.
2. Interpret the factors influencing the temperature for maximum viscosity of hollandaise sauce.
3. Outline the procedure for making a successful hollandaise sauce.

BASIC FORMULA—HOLLANDAISE SAUCE

112 g (1/2 c)	Margarine
68 g (4)	Egg yolks
60 ml (1/4 c)	Hot water
30 ml (2 tsp)	Lemon juice
1 g (1/4 tsp)	Salt

In the top part of a double boiler, melt the margarine. Remove from heat and cool to 65°C. Beat egg yolks well before stirring thoroughly into the margarine. Stir in remaining ingredients and then resume heating slowly over simmering water. Note pH. Stir continuously and watch temperature throughout the cooking period. Remove approximately 1/4 of the sauce at each of the following temperatures: 68°C, 72°C, and 76°C. If the sauce has not curdled at 76°C, continue to heat the remaining sauce until it curdles, being careful to note the final temperature.

PROCEDURE

1. **Control**—Prepare as described in the basic formula.

2. **Vinegar**—Substitute 30 ml vinegar for lemon juice and follow procedure outlined in the basic formula.

3. **Added acid**—Increase the lemon juice in the basic recipe to 60 ml and decrease hot water to 30 ml. Prepare as outlined in the basic formula.

4. **Added egg yolk**—Follow the basic formula, but increase egg yolk to a total of 102 g.

EVALUATION

1. Place samples on a hot tray or in a hot water bath to keep warm during evaluation.

CHART 7.4 HOLLANDAISE SAUCE

Treatment	pH	Appearance	Flavor	Color	Line spread
1. Control (lemon juice, citric acid) a. 68°C					XXX
b. 72°C	XXX		XXX	XXX	
c. 76°C	XXX		XXX	XXX	
2. Vinegar (acetic acid) a. 68°C					XXX
b. 72°C	XXX		XXX	XXX	
c. 76°C	XXX		XXX	XXX	
3. Added acid a. 68°C					XXX
b. 72°C	XXX		XXX	XXX	
c. 76°C	XXX		XXX	XXX	
4. Added yolk a. 68°C					XXX
b. 72°C	XXX		XXX	XXX	
c. 76°C	XXX		XXX	XXX	

Name

ADDITIONAL OBSERVATIONS AND NOTES

2. Hollandaise sauce should be a completely homogeneous, smooth, and viscous sauce with no evidence of fat separating from the emulsion. The flavor should provide a pleasing complement to vegetables and egg dishes. Subjective testing will address these criteria. The line-spread test is a useful objective test, which should be conducted when the samples are removed from the double boiler at 72°C and at 76°C.

STUDY QUESTIONS

1. At what temperature was the best sample of hollandaise sauce obtained for each of the following:

   a. Control (citric acid)?

   b. Acetic acid?

   c. Reduced pH?

   d. Increased yolk protein?

2. Discuss the role(s) of egg yolk in a hollandaise sauce.

3. What causes a hollandaise sauce to curdle? What can possibly be done to make a curdled hollandaise sauce more palatable? What precaution(s) can be taken to avoid curdling of the sauce? (Answers to ways of improving a curdled sauce can be explored by using some of the curdled sauces prepared in the experiment and attempting such techniques as stirring in hot water, stirring the sauce into a fresh egg yolk, or other techniques of interest.)

EXPERIMENT 7.5—EGG WHITE FOAMS
OBJECTIVES

Upon completion of the experiment, you will be able to:

1. Identify the factors contributing to volume of egg white foams.
2. Identify the factors contributing to stability of egg white foams.
3. Outline the method and ingredients to use in developing egg white foams of optimum volume, texture, and stability.
4. Explain the procedures to prepare a soft meringue of optimum quality for topping a cream pie.

BASIC FORMULA—EGG WHITE FOAMS

33 g (1)   Egg white

Prepare a funnel lined with filter paper by supporting it on a ring stand so that its stem drains into a 100 ml graduated cylinder.

Beat egg white in a small bowl using electric mixers of the same brand unless otherwise stated. All foams should be beaten until the peaks just bend over when the foam is pulled up with a rubber spatula. *Note the time required to beat the foam.*

With a rubber spatula, quickly and gently transfer the foam to the funnel (or to the pie filling). Insert a metal skewer vertically into the foam so that the tip of the skewer is even with the upper end of the stem of the funnel. Note the location of the uppermost part of the foam on the skewer (see Appendix A). Also measure the foam height along the funnel edge (from the stem) and average the two values. Record the drainage at 10-minute intervals for 1 hour.

PROCEDURE

1. **Type of beater**

   a. *Control, rotary beater*—Use a rotary beater to make the egg white foam, as described in the basic formula.

   b. *Wire whip*—Use a wire whip to make the egg white foam, as described in the basic formula.

   c. *Conventional electric mixer*—Use a conventional electric mixer to make the egg white foam, as described in the basic formula.

   d. *Hypocycloidal electric mixer*—Use a hypocycloidal electric mixer to make the egg white foam described in the basic formula.

2. **Addition of sugar**

   a. *1 tbsp sugar*—Prepare the basic formula, but add 12.5 g sugar gradually, beginning at the foamy stage.

b. *2 tbsp sugar*—Prepare the basic formula, but add 25 g sugar gradually, beginning at the foamy stage.

c. *3 tbsp sugar*—Prepare the basic formula, but add 37.5 g sugar gradually, beginning at the foamy stage.

d. *Sugar at beginning*—Prepare the basic formula, but add 25 g sugar before beginning to beat the meringue.

e. *Sugar at end*—Prepare basic formula, but add 25 g sugar all at once when the *peaks bend over.* Continue beating until peaks once again just bend over.

f. *Sugar folded in*—Prepare basic formula, but fold in 25 g sugar with a rubber spatula *after beating is completed.*

g. *Hot syrup*—Prepare basic formula, but use 99 g of egg white and prepare a syrup of 60 ml water and 150 g sugar that has been boiled to a temperature of 114°C (238°F). Beat the egg whites 30 seconds to form soft peaks before turning the mixer down to medium speed and slowly pouring in the syrup. Continue beating until meringue cools. Proceed with measurements as stated in the basic formula. (**Note:** this type of meringue, *Italian,* requires about 5 to 8 minutes to brown in a 425°F oven if it is being baked on a meringue pie.)

h. *Confectioners sugar*—Prepare the basic formula, but gradually add 25 g confectioners sugar, beginning at the foamy stage.

i. *Dessert (super-fine) sugar*—Prepare basic formula, but add 25 g dessert sugar gradually, beginning at the foamy stage.

j. *Honey*—Prepare the basic formula, but add 42 g (2 tbsp) honey gradually, beginning at the foamy stage.

k. *Sucralose*—Prepare the basic formula, but add 3 g sucralose (Splenda®) gradually, beginning at the foamy stage.

l. *Aspartame*—Prepare the basic formula, but add 2.4 g Equal® gradually, beginning at the foamy stage.

m. *Isomalt*—Prepare the basic formula, but add 3 g isomalt gradually, beginning at the foamy stage.

3. **Addition of acid**

a. *Citric acid*—Prepare the basic formula, but add 8 ml (1/2 tsp) lemon juice at the foamy stage.

b. *Cream of tartar*—Prepare the basic formula, but add 1.6 g (1/4 tsp) cream of tartar at the foamy stage.

c. *2x cream of tartar*—Prepare the basic formula, but add 1.6 g (1/2 tsp) cream of tartar at the foamy stage.

4. **Addition of other ingredients**

a. *Salt*—Prepare the basic formula, but add 0.8 g (1/2 tsp) salt at the foamy stage.

b. *Water*—Prepare the basic formula, but add 8 ml (1/2 tbsp) water at the foamy stage.

5. **Extent of beating**

   a. *Under-beating*—Prepare the basic formula as described, but beat the foam only until the foam can *barely* be pulled into a peak that tends to flow.

   b. *Over-beating*—Prepare the basic formula, but continue beating until the foam is dry on the surface and begins to break into pieces.

6. **Variations in beating temperatures**

   a. *Room temperature*—Prepare the basic formula, being sure the egg white is at room temperature before beginning to beat.

   b. *Refrigerator temperature*—Weigh the egg white for the basic formula. Cover tightly and refrigerate for at least 30 minutes. Remove from the refrigerator and beat *immediately*, as described in the basic formula.

7. **Baking of foams with variations in oven temperatures and pie filling temperatures** (Series to be done by 1 group.)

Prepare filling:

48 g (6 tbsp) cornstarch

200 g (1 c) sugar

944 ml (1 qt) water

Thoroughly blend the cornstarch and sugar in a saucepan. Slowly stir in the water to make a smooth slurry. Heat over direct heat, stirring constantly, until the mixture boils and becomes translucent. Pour approximately 1/8 of the mixture into each of 4 individual pie plates. Place in freezer until cooled to at least 22°C. Leave the remaining half of the filling in the pan and cover the pan.

Preheat ovens:

   a. Preheat 1 oven to 300°F (150°C)

   b. Preheat 1 oven to 350°F (177°C)

   c. Preheat 1 oven to 400°F (205°C)

   d. Preheat 1 oven to 450°F (232°C)

Prepare meringue:

180 g (6) egg whites

4.8 g (1 1/2 tsp) cream of tartar

150 g (3/4 c) sugar

Beat egg whites on fastest speed of conventional electric mixer until foamy. Add all of the cream of tartar and begin to add the sugar gradually. Continue beating until peaks bend over when pulled up with a rubber spatula.

Assembly of meringue experiment:

Place the refrigerated samples on the counter. Bring the remaining filling in the pan to a boil and quickly pour into the remaining 4 individual pie plates. Immediately place 1/8 of the meringue on each pie, being careful to seal the meringue to the edge of the plates.

Baking:

Place 1 of the cold filling and 1 of the hot filling pies in an oven preheated to (a) 300°F; similarly, place 1 of the cold and 1 of the hot filling pies in (b) the 350°F oven, (c) the 400°F, and (d) the 450°F oven. Bake the meringues in each oven to the same golden brown color. Note the time required to reach this point in each oven. Cool at least 10 minutes before beginning evaluation.

EVALUATION

1. The unbaked egg white foams should be evaluated on the basis of their volume (as indicated by the height of the foam), their texture (as assessed visually), and by their stability (as indicated by the amount of drainage). The time required to form the foam indicates the relative ease of formation and is of particular interest if foams are to be beaten by hand.

2. Baked meringues are evaluated on the basis of their volume after baking, their tendency to shrink from the edge of the pan, the texture, surface appearance, and stability. Subjective measures are used. The pies should be judged for appearance before the meringues are cut.

   Ease of cutting can be evaluated by making a single cut with all students watching. The meringue should not cling to the knife. Volume can be estimated by looking at a cross section of the meringue after a section has been removed. Of particular interest is the amount of drainage that occurs upon standing. If possible, pies should be allowed to stand at least an hour, at which time the plates can be tipped to collect any drainage at one side.

STUDY QUESTIONS

1. What factors contribute to making an egg white foam with a large volume?

2. What factors contribute to the stability of an egg white foam?

3. Which type of beater resulted in the foam with the largest volume? The greatest stability?

4. At what level does sugar provide optimal volume to an egg white foam? Maximum stability?

5. How did the higher sugar level and heat of the syrup affect the egg white foam? Explain why these changes occurred.

6. Describe the changes in egg white foams when the following are added: (a) confectioners sugar, (b) dessert sugar, (c) honey, (d) aspartame, (e) sucralose, and (f) isomalt.

7. Compare the stability achieved by the addition of lemon juice to an egg white foam with that achieved by the addition of cream of tartar (tartaric acid) at 2 different levels.

8. What is the effect of added salt on stability of an egg white foam? On volume?

9. What is the effect of added water on stability of an egg white foam? On volume?

10. Describe the changes in volume and stability of egg white foams as the extent of beating is increased.

11. Compare the ease of foam formation, the volume, and the stability of foams made from the whites of fresh, frozen, and deteriorated eggs.

12. How does the temperature of the whites influence egg white foams?

13. Describe the conditions that will result in an optimum meringue on a pie.

CHART 7.5 EGG WHITE FOAMS

Treatment	Time (min)	Volume mean ht. (mm)	Texture	Drainage (ml)					
				10 (min.)	20 (min.)	30 (min.)	40 (min.)	50 (min.)	60 (min.)
1. Beater									
a. Rotary*									
b. Whip									
c. Conv. el.									
d. Hypo. el.									
2. Sugar									
a. 1 tbsp									
b. 2 tbsp									
c. 3 tbsp									
d. Beginning									
e. End									
f. Fold									
g. Hot syrup									
h. Confectioners									
i. Dessert									
j. Honey									
k. Sucralose (Splenda®)									
l. Aspartame (Equal®)									
m. Isomalt									
3. Acid									
a. 1/2 tsp lemon juice									
b. 1/4 tsp cr. tartar									
c. 1/2 tsp cr. tartar									
4. Other ingredients									
a. Salt									
b. Water									
5. Beating									
a. Underbeaten									
b. Overbeaten									
6. Temp.									
a. Room									
b. Refrig.									

* Control

Name

ADDITIONAL OBSERVATIONS AND NOTES

CHART 7.5   EGG WHITE FOAMS (CONTINUED)

Treatment	Time (min)	Volume mean ht. (mm)	Texture	Drainage (ml)					
				10 (min.)	20 (min.)	30 (min.)	40 (min.)	50 (min.)	60 (min.)
7. Baked, hot fill.									
a. 150°C (300°F)				XXX	XXX	XXX	XXX	XXX	XXX
b. 177°C (350°F)				XXX	XXX	XXX	XXX	XXX	XXX
c. 205°C (400°F)				XXX	XXX	XXX	XXX	XXX	XXX
d. 232°C (450°F)				XXX	XXX	XXX	XXX	XXX	XXX
8. Baked, cold fill.									
a. 150°C (300°F)				XXX	XXX	XXX	XXX	XXX	XXX
b. 177°C (350°F)				XXX	XXX	XXX	XXX	XXX	XXX
c. 205°C (400°F)				XXX	XXX	XXX	XXX	XXX	XXX
d. 232°C (450°F)				XXX	XXX	XXX	XXX	XXX	XXX

Name

ADDITIONAL OBSERVATIONS AND NOTES

EXPERIMENT 7.6—ANGEL CAKES
OBJECTIVES

Upon completion of the experiment, you will be able to:

1. Outline the best method for making an angel cake with optimum texture, volume, and tenderness.
2. Evaluate angel cakes according to accepted standards.
3. Relate the effect of mixing to the texture, volume, and tenderness of angel cake.
4. Explain the role of cream of tartar in an angel cake.
5. Interpret the effect of sugar on flavor, tenderness, volume, and texture of angel cake.
6. Describe the interrelationship of sugar (or alternative sweetener) and gluten development in angel cake.
7. Relate the effect of foam development on texture, volume, and tenderness of angel cakes.
8. Explain the influence of baking conditions in determining quality of angel cake.
9. Compare the merits of all purpose and cake flour in preparation of angel cake.

BASIC FORMULA—ANGEL CAKE

10 g	Sugar
15 g	Cake flour
41 g	Egg whites
32 g	Sugar
0.6 g	Cream of tartar
0.1 g	Salt

Preheat oven to 350°F (177°C) except for procedure 6, which has separate baking directions.

Line the bottom of each individual loaf pan (5" × 2 1/2" × 2") with wax paper cut to just fit. Do *not* grease the sides of the pan.

Sift flour and first weight (10 g) of sugar together and set aside. Beat the egg whites together to the foamy stage, using an electric mixer (same kind for all parts of the experiment). Unless indicated differently in a specific series, add the cream of tartar and salt. (**Note:** if it were being used, flavoring would be added with the cream of tartar.) Continue beating on the fastest mixer setting while gradually adding 32 g sugar. Beat the whites until the peaks just bend over. Sift 1/4 of the flour-sugar mixture over the whites. Fold in gently with 10 strokes using a rubber spatula. Sift the second 1/4 of the flour-sugar mixture over the whites and fold in gently with 10 strokes, followed by the same process for the third addition. Sift the final 1/4 of the flour-sugar mixture over the foam and fold 20 strokes to completely blend the mixture (making a total of 50 folding strokes with the rubber spatula). Gently push and weigh 99 g of the batter into the pan. Finish all of the cakes being baked in one oven before placing them all in the oven at the same time. Bake until the surface springs back when touched lightly with a finger (~30 minutes). Record the baking time. Cool in an inverted position with air circulating under the pan. When almost cool, remove from the pan.

PROCEDURE

1. **Varying the amount of folding**

   a. *20 strokes*—Follow the basic formula, but fold only 5 strokes after each addition (a total of 20 strokes).

   b. *50 strokes (control)*—Follow the basic formula.

   c. *80 strokes*—Follow the basic formula, but fold 20 strokes after each addition (a total of 80 strokes).

2. **Varying the amount of beating of the whites**

   a. *Under-beating*—Prepare the basic formula, but beat the whites only to the point where they will *not quite* hold a peak.

   b. *Over-beating*—Prepare the basic formula, but beat the whites until they are brittle and dry.

3. **Varying cream of tartar**

   a. *No cream of tartar*—Prepare the basic formula, but omit the cream of tartar.

   b. *Double cream of tartar*—Prepare the basic formula, but use double (1.2 g) cream of tartar.

4. **Varying the amount and type of flour**

   a. *All purpose flour*—Prepare the basic formula, but use all purpose flour in place of cake flour.

   b. *Decreased cake flour*—Prepare the basic formula, but decrease cake flour to a total of 10 g.

   c. *Increased cake flour*—Prepare the basic formula, but increase cake flour to a total of 20 g.

   d. *Cornstarch*—Prepare the basic formula, but omit cake flour and replace with 15 g of corn starch.

5. **Varying sugar**

   a. *Reduced sugar*—Prepare the basic formula, but use only 8 g for the first sugar weight and only 26 g sugar for the second weight.

   b. *Increased sugar*—Prepare the basic formula, but use 13 g sugar for the first weight and 38 g sugar for the second weight.

   c. *Excess sugar*—Prepare the basic formula, but use 17 g for the first weight of sugar and 50 g for the second weight.

   d. *Sugar replacement (sucralose)*—Prepare the basic formula, but omit sugar and use 1.2 g sucralose for the first weight of sugar and 1.2 g sucralose for the second weight of sugar.

   e. *Sugar replacement (isomalt)*—Prepare the basic formula, but omit sugar and use 1.8 g isomalt for the first weight of sugar and 1.8 g isomalt for the second weight of sugar.

6. **Varying baking conditions**—Batter for all 6 cakes is prepared in a single batch (see cake preparation instructions below) and then 1 is baked in each of the following treatments:

a. *Cold*—No preheating. Turn on oven set to 350°F (177°C) when cake is placed in the oven.

b. *325°F (163°C)*—Preheat oven to temperature before placing cake in the oven.

c. *350°F (177°C)*—Preheat oven to temperature before placing the cake in the oven.

d. *375°F (190°C)*—Preheat oven to temperature before placing the cake in the oven.

e. *400°F (205°C)*—Preheat oven to temperature before placing the cake in the oven.

f. *450°F (232°C)*—Preheat oven to temperature before placing cake in the oven.

Cake preparation instructions: Sift together 60 g sugar and 90 g cake flour. Beat 244 g egg white until foamy. Add 3.6 g cream of tartar and 1 g salt. Gradually begin adding 190 g sugar while beating on fastest speed until peaks just bend over. Add the sugar-flour mixture in 4 additions, as described in the basic formula. Weigh 99 g of batter into each of 6 individual loaf pans. Place 1 cake in each of the ovens prepared for variations a–f above. Bake each until the top of the cake springs back when touched lightly with a finger. Carefully note and record the baking time for each of the variations. Cool as described in the basic formula.

EVALUATION

Objective evaluation   After cooling, carefully wrap each cake in plastic wrap and use the volumeter to determine the volume of each cake. If a volumeter is not available, a seed displacement device can be constructed or an inkblot can be made of the cross section of the center of the cake. The inkblot can be traced by a planimeter to determine the area of the cross section. The inkblot serves as a permanent record of the texture of the cake, as well as providing a standard for determining relative volume of the cakes.

Subjective evaluation   Evaluation of the exterior includes judging the general conformation of the cake, its surface appearance and browning characteristics. The interior texture should be examined for size and uniformity of cells and thickness of cell walls. Whiteness of the crumb can be determined visually, too. Tenderness can be assessed by counting the number of chews required for chewing a sample of defined size to a specific end point. The "number of chews" test is done for each sample. Flavor also should be noted.

STUDY QUESTIONS

1. Describe the desired characteristics of an angel cake of excellent quality.

2. What effect can be noted as the amount of mixing is increased during the folding of the flour-sugar mixture into the egg white foam? Why would one predict this effect?

3. Compare the characteristics of angel cakes made with whites that are (a) underbeaten, (b) beaten correctly, and (c) overbeaten.

4. Describe the changes that can be noted when the level of cream of tartar varies from none to double the normal amount. Does the cream of tartar have a comparable effect when it is added with the flour rather than being beaten into the egg white foam? Explain.

5. What is the effect of (a) reducing the amount of cake flour, (b) increasing the amount of cake flour, and (c) substituting all purpose flour in making angel cakes?

6. Describe the change(s) that can be observed when the level of sugar in angel cake is increased gradually. Does this increase have any influence on the amount of folding required for adding the flour-sugar mixture? Why?

7. Compare the control cake in 1b (made with sugar) with cakes made with (a) sucralose and (b) isomalt. Explain why these results occurred.

8. Is it necessary to preheat an oven to achieve optimum quality in an angel cake? What oven temperature is best for baking an angel cake?

CHART 7.6   ANGEL CAKES

Treatment	Baking time	Volume	Exterior		Texture of crumb	Tenderness (# chews)	Comments
			Color	Shape			
1. Folding							
a. 20x							
b. 50x*							
c. 80x							
2. Beating							
a. Under							
b. Over							
3. Cream of tartar							
a. None							
b. 2x							
4. Flour							
a. All purpose							
b. 66% cake							
c. 133% cake							
d. Cornstarch							
5. Sugar							
a. 80% sugar							
b. 120% sugar							
c. 162% sugar							
d. Sucralose							
e. Isomalt							
6. Baking							
a. No preheat 350°C (177°F)							
b. 325°F (163°C) preheat							
c. 350°F (177°C) preheat							
d. 375°F (190°C) preheat							
e. 400°F (205°C) preheat							
f. 450°F (232°C) preheat							

*Control

Name

ADDITIONAL OBSERVATIONS AND NOTES

8

Leavening Agents

Air, steam, and carbon dioxide are the source of leavening in baked products. As batters and doughs are mixed, some air always will be incorporated into the mixture. Also, there always is some water present. When the batter or dough is heated in the oven, the air begins to expand and exert pressure against the cell walls. Similarly, water eventually is converted to steam during baking, and the steam exerts significant pressure on cell walls. If baking powder, yeast, or a combination of acidic and alkaline ingredients is present, carbon dioxide will be generated in the product. This gas also expands during baking of the food. The pressure exerted by air, steam, and/or carbon dioxide is capable of stretching cell walls as long as the proteins of the cell walls are not denatured. When gluten or egg proteins are denatured, they no longer are capable of stretching, and the final structure is set.

The optimal circumstance for leavening most baked products is to incorporate some air uniformly throughout the batter or dough during mixing. This is followed by additional gas being generated during the early baking period. The additional gas is very effective in helping to stretch the structure and maintain adequate pressure until the protein denatures and the structure is set. However, too much pressure from leavening agents can strain cell walls to the point that they rupture, and the product falls.

The experiments in this chapter are designed to demonstrate the mode of operation of the various types of leavening agents, the conditions required for their reactions, and the results of varying bench time and baking temperatures.

EXPERIMENT 8.1—YEAST
OBJECTIVES

Upon completion of the experiment, you will be able to:

1. Outline the optimum physical conditions for producing yeast-leavened products and predict the consequences of variations in mixing, proofing, baking temperatures, and formula modifications.
2. Discuss the reasons for the conditions that are recommended for producing leavening in yeast-containing products.
3. Use ink blots or photo copying as a technique for assessing texture of baked products.

BASIC FORMULA—BREAD

200 g (1 7/8 c)	All purpose flour
7 g (1 package)	Dry yeast
6 g (11 1/2 tsp)	Sugar
1.5 g (1/4 tsp)	Salt
118 ml (1/2 c)	Water (35°C)
4 g (1 tsp)	Shortening

Add yeast to half (59 ml) of the water after being certain the water temperature is 35°C (95°F). Barely melt the shortening. Place the sugar, salt, and other half of the water in a mixing bowl. Add the yeast-water mixture. Stir to blend. Gradually begin to add the flour while mixing slowly with an electric mixer.

Add just enough flour to make a very soft paste. Beat with the electric mixer until smooth. Remove beater blades and scrape them thoroughly with a rubber spatula to avoid losing any dough. Continue mixing by hand with a wooden spoon. Add just enough flour to make a smooth, non-sticky, rather soft dough. If all of the weighed flour is used, weigh another 25 g and use what is needed to make the dough manageable. Knead the dough with the heel of the hands on a board floured very lightly with some of the weighed flour. Knead by folding the far edge of the dough to meet the front edge, pushing firmly with the heels of both hands, and rotating 90°. Continue the pattern of folding, pushing, and rotating 90° until 100 kneading strokes have been completed.

Very lightly coat the dough ball with oil. Place in a beaker large enough to hold the dough when it has doubled in size; cover with aluminum foil. Let rise 30 minutes in a water bath maintained at 32°C (90°F). Estimate the volume of the risen dough. Punch dough down. Shape into a loaf and place in a loaf pan that has been greased on the bottom. Return to the water bath and let rise until double in volume. Meanwhile preheat oven to 220°C (425°F). Note time required for the second rising to double the volume. Bake in the center of the oven at 220°C for about 15 minutes (until the bread sounds hollow when the top is tapped). Measure volume. Remove from the pan. Cool on a wire rack.

PROCEDURE

1. **Variations in yeast**—Prepare 3 times the basic formula. Divide into 3 equal amounts, using 1 for each of the following 3 baking temperature variations (a1, a2, and a3).

   a. *Baking temperature*

      1. **Bake at 220°C (425°F)**—Bake 1 loaf according to the basic formula. This is the control.

      2. **Bake at 175°C (350°F)**—Bake 1 loaf at 175°C.

      3. **Bake at 150°C (300°F)**—Bake 1 loaf at 150°C.

   b. *Dry yeast halved*—Prepare basic formula, but use 3.5 g yeast.

   c. *Dry yeast doubled*—Prepare basic formula, but use 14 g yeast.

   d. *Compressed yeast*—Prepare basic formula, but use 15.75 g compressed yeast. (This is equivalent to 7 g dry yeast.)

2. **Variations in ingredients**

   a. *0 g sugar*—Prepare basic formula, but omit the sugar.

   b. *Sugar (control)*—Prepare basic formula with the normal level of 6 g of sugar, or use sample 1a1 as the control.

   c. *Sugar doubled*—Prepare basic formula, but use 12 g of sugar.

   d. *0 g salt*—Prepare basic formula, but omit the salt.

   e. *Salt (control)*—Prepare basic formula with normal level of 1.5 g salt or use sample 1a1 as the control.

   f. *Salt doubled*—Prepare basic formula, but use 3 g salt.

3. **Variations in proofing temperatures**

   a. *Proof at 24°C (75°F)*—Prepare basic formula, but control the water bath temperature at 24°C for both rising periods.

   b. *Proof at 28°C (82°F)*—Prepare the basic formula, but control the water bath temperature at 28°C for both rising periods.

   c. *Proof at 32°C (90°F)*—Use sample 1a1 as the control or prepare the basic formula, and control the water bath temperature at 32°C for both rising periods.

   d. *Proof at 40°C (104°F)*—Prepare the basic formula, but control the water bath at 40°C for both rising periods.

EVALUATION

Note the estimated volumes for the first rising period and the time required during the second proofing period to achieve a doubling of volume. Determine the volume of the baked bread by using a volumeter or by filling the baking pan containing the bread with rape seeds, measuring the volume of seeds required to fill the pan, and then subtracting the seed volume from the total volume of the pan. After the bread has cooled at least 10 minutes on a wire rack, slice the loaf in half and remove a center cross-sectional slice at least 1/2" thick. Photocopy this or press this slice on an inkpad and then make a print on a sheet of paper. This process should give a complete picture of the outline of the slice and a relatively clear picture of the texture. Also, evaluate the bread subjectively. Note the color, shape, and smoothness of the crust, and evaluate the flavor, tenderness, moistness, and texture of the interior.

STUDY QUESTIONS

1. What is the result when yeast produces too little carbon dioxide prior to placing the bread in the oven?

2. If yeast is softened in water at a temperature of 65°C (150°F) and then incorporated in a dough that is proofed at 24°C (75°F), what will be the characteristics of the bread made from the dough?

3. What effect does sugar have on carbon dioxide formation by yeast? What is the effect of salt on yeast?

4. Compare the advantages and disadvantages of using dry and compressed yeasts. Do they leaven by the same reaction?

5. Is it more important to control the extent of rising in the second rising than in the first rising period? Explain your answer.

6. If no proofing time is allowed, what will be the result in a yeast-leavened bread?

CHART 8.1 YEAST

Treatment	Volume 1st rising	Time of 2nd rising	Loaf volume (ml)
1. Yeast 1.a. Baking temp. 1.a.1. 220°C*			
1.a.2. 175°C			
1.a.3. 150°C			
1.b. Dry yeast, 3.5 g			
Dry yeast, 7 g* (see 1.a.1)			
1.c. Dry yeast, 14 g			
1.d. Compressed yeast			
2. Ingredients a. 0 g sugar			
b. 6 g sugar* (see 1.a.1)			
c. 12 g sugar			
d. 0 g salt			
e. 1.5 g salt* (see 1.a.1)			
f. 3 g salt			
3. Proofing temperature a. 24°C			
b. 28°C			
c. 32°C* (see 1.a.1)			
d. 40°C			

*Control

Name

ADDITIONAL OBSERVATIONS AND NOTES

CHART 8.1 YEAST (CONTINUED)

Treatment	Crust			Interior			
	Color	Shape	Smoothness	Flavor	Moistness	Tenderness	Texture
1.Yeast 1.a. Baking temp. 1.a.1. 220°C*							
1.a.2. 175°C							
1.a. 3. 150°C							
1.b. Dry yeast, 3.5 g							
Dry yeast, 7 g* (see 1.a.1)							
1.c. Dry yeast, 14 g							
1.d. Compressed yeast							
2. Ingredients a. 0 g sugar							
b. 6 g sugar* (see 1.a.1)							
c. 12 g sugar							
d. 0 g salt							
e. 1.5 g salt* (see 1.a.1)							
f. 3 g salt							
3. Proofing temperature a. 24°C							
b. 28°C* (see 1.a.1)							
c. 32°C* (see 1.a.1)							
d. 40°C							

_____ *Control

Name

ADDITIONAL OBSERVATIONS AND NOTES

EXPERIMENT 8.2—CHEMICAL REACTIONS
OBJECTIVES

Upon completion of the experiment, you will be able to:

1. Explain the role of each of the ingredients in commercial baking powders.
2. Analyze a recipe for leavening agents and determine the importance of speed in initiating baking of the product (based on the type of leavening agent used).
3. Discuss the advantages and disadvantages of the various chemical leavening agents that are available for use in the home.

BASIC FORMULA—LEAVENING

16 g	Egg white
118 ml	Water (or assigned liquid)

Egg whites
(Egg whites for the entire class are prepared by very slightly beating 6 egg whites together.)
   Weigh out 16 g for each variation to be performed. Blend the 16 g of egg white by beating it slightly with 118 ml of the liquid stated for the variation being prepared. Use water unless another liquid is stated.

Dry ingredients
Place the dry ingredient(s) assigned in the bottom of a *dry* 250 ml graduated cylinder. When all members of the class are ready, one person will give the signal for all people simultaneously to pour the egg white liquid into the cylinder immediately. Shake the cylinder just enough to ensure that all of the dry ingredients are moistened thoroughly. At the end of 30 seconds, the timer signals for the volume at the top of the foam in the cylinder to be read and recorded. The timer again gives the signal at the end of the next 30 seconds (1 minute total elapsed time) for the volume to be read again in the same way. Similarly, the timer continues to call for readings at the end of the second, third, fourth, fifth, and sixth minutes. At the end of 6 minutes, the reading is taken and the timer signals for the cylinders containing the foams to be placed in pans of water, which are heated to boiling during the first part of the experiment. The timer calls for reading the volume at the end of 30 seconds, 60 seconds, and 2, 3, 4, and 5 minutes.

PROCEDURE

1. **Leavening agents**

   a. *Baking soda*—Use 2 g baking soda as the dry ingredient in the experiment.

   b. *Baking soda and cream of tartar*—Mix 2.75 g cream of tartar and 1.1 g baking soda together very thoroughly and use as the dry ingredient in the experiment.

c. *Homemade tartrate baking powder*—Mix 1.1 g baking soda, 0.8 g cornstarch, and 2.1 g cream of tartar together very thoroughly. From this mixture weigh out 2 g and use this as the dry ingredient in the experiment.

d. *Baking soda and sour milk*—Place 2 g baking soda in the graduated cylinder to use as the dry ingredient in the experiment. Use sour milk for the liquid added to the egg white.

e. *Baking soda and molasses*—Place 2 g baking soda in the graduated cylinder. In a beaker, blend together 59 ml molasses and 59 ml water to serve as the liquid to be added to the egg white in this experiment.

f. *Baking soda and honey*—Place 2 g baking soda in the graduated cylinder. In a beaker, blend together 59 ml honey and 59 ml water to serve as the liquid to be added to the egg white.

g. *Tartrate baking powder*—Use 1.9 g tartrate baking powder, such as Royal baking powder, as the dry ingredient in the experiment.

h. *Double-acting baking powder*—Use 1.8 g double-acting baking powder, such as Calumet, as the dry ingredient in the experiment.

i. *Other baking powder*—Use 1.8 g of another double-acting baking powder (such as Clabber Girl) or 2.2 g if the powder is a phosphate baking powder.

j. *Additional checks*—If additional students are available, repeat as many of the previous variations as possible. (**Note:** additional whites will be needed.)

EVALUATION

This experiment is geared to demonstrate the production of carbon dioxide at room and at elevated temperatures. The speed of reaction is important because of its influence on the selection of a method for combining ingredients, as well as on baking conditions. Accurate readings of volume at precisely the time called out by the timer are essential to the results of this experiment. Particular attention should be directed to the amount of gas generated in the latter part of the experiment because continued production of gas during the early part of baking improves the volume of chemically leavened baked products.

STUDY QUESTIONS

1. What are the essential ingredients for carbon dioxide to be produced in a recipe?

2. What are the normal ingredients in baking powders manufactured for the retail market?

CHART 8.2 RATE OF CARBON DIOXIDE PRODUCTION BY VARIOUS CHEMICALS

Treatment	Volume (room temp.)							Volume (temp. boiling water bath)					
	30 sec.	1 min.	2 min.	3 min.	4 min.	5 min.	6 min.	30 min.	1 min.	2 min.	3 min.	4 min.	5 min.
a. Baking soda													
b. Baking soda + cr. tartar													
c. Homemade tartrate b.p.													
d. Baking soda + sour milk													
e. Baking soda + molasses													
f. Baking soda + honey													
g. Tartrate, b.p. Brand: _____													
h. Double-acting baking powder Brand: ____													
i. Other type: _____ Brand: _____													

Name

ADDITIONAL OBSERVATIONS AND NOTES

3. What are the advantages of using a commercial baking powder compared with using sour milk and soda?

4. What are the advantages and disadvantages of the various types of commercial baking powders presently marketed for home use?

5. Why is there a federal regulation regarding the minimum level of carbon dioxide production that must be provided by a baking powder?

6. Compare the gas production from the combination of soda with each of the following: (a) sour milk, (b) molasses, (c) honey, and (d) cream of tartar.

7. When should the soda be added if a product is to be leavened by soda and sour milk? Why? Would you recommend this recipe to someone who is just learning to cook? Why? Should the oven be preheated? Why?

EXPERIMENT 8.3—USE OF NON-BIOLOGICAL LEAVENING AGENTS OBJECTIVES

Upon completion of the experiment, you will be able to:

1. Interpret the role of air, steam, and carbon dioxide from chemical reactions as leavening agents.
2. Evaluate the importance of rapid baking of products leavened with air, steam, and/or chemical leaveners.
3. Assess potential flavor and color contributions of leavening agents.
4. Identify the ingredients in a recipe that will contribute to the leavening of the product and recommend ways of combining ingredients and of baking the product to optimize volume.

BASIC FORMULA—POPOVERS (EXPERIMENT 8.3.1)

Full batch		Half batch
236 ml (1 c)	Milk	118 ml (1/2 c)
96 g (2)	Eggs	48 g (1)
110 g (1c)	Flour	58 g (1/2 c)
3 g (1/2 tsp)	Salt	1.5 g (1/4 tsp)

Lightly grease custard cups and place in the oven while it is preheating to 425°F (220°C) and the batter is being prepared.

Combine the milk, eggs, flour, and salt in the small bowl of an electric mixer. Rotate the bowl (with the beater blades immersed) just enough to dampen the flour. Turn the electric mixer to the highest speed for 1 minute. Measure 50 ml batter and quickly pour into a preheated custard cup. Bake at 425°F for 40 minutes. Puncture with a 2-tined kitchen fork and continue baking 5 more minutes. Remove from custard cups immediately.

PROCEDURE

1. **Conditions prior to baking**—(**Note:** 3 variations are done by 1 group.) Prepare a *full* batch, following the basic formula. Preheat 2 greased cups in 425°F oven and have the other 4 cups greased and ready on the counter. Prepare 2 popovers by each of the following treatments.

   a. *Start in cold cups*—Pour 50 ml of batter into each of 2 greased cups. Set together on counter. These then will be placed on the jelly roll pan with the 2 popovers being prepared in 1c and baked at 220°C (425°F).

   b. *Bench time of 30 minutes in cups*—Pour 50 ml of the batter into each of 2 greased (cold) cups and let them sit on the counter for 30 minutes. Then bake in a preheated oven at 220°C (425°F) according to the basic formula.

   c. *Start in hot cups (control)*—Pour 50 ml of the batter into each of the 2 preheated cups (removed from the oven using hot pads right before the batter is poured). Place on the jelly roll pan with the 2 cups from 1a and bake immediately at 220°C as described in the basic formula.

2. **Conditions during baking**

   a. *No preheating, 220°C bake*—Prepare a *half* batch according to the basic formula. Pour 50 ml batter into each of 3 greased, cold custard cups. Place on a jelly roll pan in a cold oven. Immediately turn the oven on to a setting of 425°F (220°C) and bake according to the formula instructions.

   b. *Preheated oven, 177°C (350°F)*—Prepare *half* a batch following the basic formula; pour 50 ml batter into each of 3 greased, preheated custard cups that were heated on a jelly roll pan at 177°C. Immediately place the cups in the oven at 177°C and bake according to the basic formula.

   c. *Preheated oven, 204°C (400°F)*—Prepare *half* a batch following the basic formula. Pour 509 ml batter into each of 3 custard cups that have been preheated on a jelly roll pan in an oven at 204°C. Bake according to the basic formula, but at 204°C.

   d. *Preheated oven, 220°C (425°F) (control)*—Prepare *half* a batch following the basic formula. Pour 50 ml batter into each of 3 custard cups preheated on a jelly roll pan in an oven at 218°C (425°F). Bake as in the basic formula.

   e. *Preheated oven, 232°C (450°F)*—Prepare *half* a batch following the basic formula. Pour 50 ml batter into each of 3 custard cups that have been preheated on a jelly roll pan in an oven at 232°C. Bake according to the basic formula, but at 232°C (450°F).

EVALUATION

Determine the volume of the largest popover from each variation. After the volume has been measured, this popover can be put on display whole for all students to evaluate for external appearance. The remainder of the popovers from each variation can be broken open to assess the openness of the cavity. Sensory evaluation should include the crispness of the shell of the popover, external appearance, and flavor.

CHART 8.3.1   STEAM AS A LEAVENING AGENT—POPOVERS

Treatment	Volume		Appearance		Shell crispness	Flavor
	Final	% Increase*	Exterior	Cavity		
1. Prior to baking at 220°C a. Cold cups						
b. 30 min. bench						
c. Hot cups (control)						
2. During baking a. No preheat, 220°C						
b. Preheat, 177°C						
c. Preheat, 204°C						
d. Preheat, 220°C						
e. Preheat, 232°C						

$$*\% \text{ increase} = \frac{\text{final volume in ml} - 50 \text{ ml}}{50 \text{ ml}} \times 100$$

Note: 50 ml was the original volume prior to baking.

ADDITIONAL OBSERVATIONS AND NOTES

BASIC FORMULA—ANGEL CAKE (EXPERIMENT 8.3.2)

30 g	Sugar
45 g	Cake flour
123 g	Egg whites
96 g	Sugar
1.8 g	Cream of tartar
0.3 g	Salt

Preheat ovens according to variations below. Line 3 pans (5 × 2 1/2 × 2 1/2 inches) with wax paper cut to just fit the bottom of each pan. Sift flour and the first weight (30 g) of sugar together and set aside. Beat the egg whites to the foamy stage, using an electric mixer set at top speed. Add the cream of tartar and salt. Resume beating on top speed while gradually adding the remaining 96 g of sugar. Beat the whites until the peaks just bend over. Sift 1/4 of the flour-sugar mixture over the whites. Fold in gently with 10 strokes of a rubber spatula. Sift the second 1/4 of the flour-sugar mixture over the foam and fold in gently with another 10 strokes, followed by the third addition and another 10 folding strokes. Finally, sift the last 1/4 of the flour-sugar mixture over the foam and fold 20 strokes to completely blend the mixture (making a total of 50 strokes). Divide the batter into the 3 pans (85 g in each). Use a wax pencil to mark the level of the batter on the outside of each pan. Bake, according to the directions in the variations, until the cake springs back when touched lightly with a finger.

After baking, cool in an inverted position with air circulating under the pan. When cool, remove from pans.

PROCEDURE

3. **Baking conditions for angel cake**—These 3 variations are done by 1 group.

   a. *30 minutes bench time*—Let 1 cake sit on the bench for 30 minutes before baking in a preheated oven at 177°C (350°F) until done (~30 minutes). Note baking time.

   b. *Preheated oven, 177°C (350°F)*—Place 1 cake immediately in a preheated oven and bake at 177°C until done. Note baking time.

   c. *Preheated oven, 218°C (425°F)*—Place 1 cake immediately in a preheated oven and bake at 218°C until done. Note baking time.

EVALUATION

Before removing angel cake from the pan, let it cool thoroughly. Measure the volume in the volumeter. (Original batter volume equals the volume of water required to fill the pan to the level marked on it before baking).

CHART 8.3.2   AIR AS A LEAVENING AGENT—ANGEL CAKE

Treatment	Volume				Texture		Tender-ness	Comments
	Original (ml)	Final (ml)	Difference (ml)	% increase of cells*	Size	Uniformity		
a. 30 minutes bench								
b. Preheated, 177°C (control)								
c. Preheated, 218°C								

$$*\% \text{ increase} = \frac{\text{final volume in ml } - \text{ original volume in ml}}{\text{original volume in ml}} \times 100$$

ADDITIONAL OBSERVATIONS AND NOTES

BASIC FORMULA—GINGERBREAD (EXPERIMENT 8.3.3)

3x (variation 4)

59 ml (1/4 c)	Molasses	177 ml (3/4 c)
30 ml (2 tbsp)	Sour milk*	90 ml (6 tbsp)
15 ml (1 tbsp)	Corn oil	45 ml (3 tbsp)
12 g (1/4)	Egg	36 g (3/4)
55 g (1/2 c)	Flour, all purpose	165 g (1 1/2 c)
2 g (1/2 tsp)	Soda	6 g (1 1/2 tsp)
0.9 g (3/8 tsp)	Ginger	2.7 g (1 1/8 tsp)
0.75 g (1/8 tsp)	Salt	2.2 g (1 1/8 tsp)

Optional: inclusion of spices may interfere with flavor evaluation

0.3 g (1/8 tsp)	Cloves	0.9 g (3/8 tsp)
0.3 g (1/8 tsp)	Mace	0.9 g (3/8 tsp)
0.6 g (1/4 tsp)	Cinnamon	1.8 g (3/4 tsp)
0.6 g (1/4 tsp)	Allspice	1.8 g (3/4 tsp)

*Sour milk by letting it stand for 10 minutes after adding lemon juice (2 ml juice and 38 ml milk for the small formula, 6 ml juice and 84 ml milk for the large).

Preheat oven to 185°C (365°F). Place all ingredients in a mixing bowl and beat 100 strokes with a wooden spoon. Check the pH of the batter quickly. Pour 160 g of batter into a loaf pan (5 3/4″ × 3 1/2″ × 2″). With a wax marking pencil, mark the outside of the pan to show the level of the batter. Bake at 185°C (365°F) until a toothpick inserted in center comes out clean. Note baking time. Cool in an upright position before removing from the pan for evaluation.

PROCEDURE

4. **Baking conditions for gingerbread**—(**Note:** All variations are done by 1 group.) Prepare *3 times* the basic gingerbread formula; weigh 160 g of batter into each of 3 pans. Bake one according to each of the following methods. Be sure to use a wax pencil to mark the outside of the baking pan to show the level of the batter prior to baking. Cool the cakes in an upright position before removing from the pans for evaluation.

   a. *30 minutes bench time*—Let the batter stand in the pan 30 minutes before baking according to the basic formula.

   b. *Control*—Bake as stated in the basic formula.

   c. *No preheating*—Place one cake in a cold oven. Immediately begin heating the oven to 185°C (365°F).

5. **Variations in leavening**

   a. *Sweet milk and some baking powder*—Prepare basic gingerbread formula, but use 30 ml *sweet* milk, reduce soda to 1 g and add 2.7 g double-acting baking powder. Follow directions in the basic formula. Check the pH of the batter very quickly. Do not delay baking.

b. *Sweet milk*—Prepare the basic gingerbread formula, but substitute 30 ml sweet milk for the 30 ml sour milk.

EVALUATION

The original volume of the batter and the final volume of the baked product should be determined, as described for angel cake. Determine the difference in volume between the batter and the baked product. Be sure to record the pH of all of the gingerbread batters. Sensory evaluation of gingerbread should include visual assessment of the color and an attempt to correlate the color with the pH measurements. In addition to color, evaluate for texture, tenderness, and flavor. In evaluating flavor, be sure to exhale sharply after swallowing to detect any flavor overtones.

CHART 8.3.3   CHEMICAL LEAVENING AGENTS—GINGERBREAD

Treatment	Volume			pH	Color	Texture	Tenderness	Flavor
	Original (ml)	Final (ml)	% increase*					
4. Baking a. 30 min. bench								
b. 185°C (control)								
c. No preheat								
5. Variation in leavening a. Sweet milk + b.p.								
b. Sweet milk								

$$*\% \text{ increase} = \frac{\text{final volume in ml} - \text{original volume in ml}}{\text{original volume in ml}} \times 100$$

Name

ADDITIONAL OBSERVATIONS AND NOTES

BASIC FORMULA—BISCUITS (EXPERIMENT 8.3.4)

116 g (1 c)	All purpose flour
5.4 g (1 1/2 tsp)	Baking powder (double-acting)
1.5 g (1/4 tsp)	Salt
24 g (2 tbsp)	Shortening
95 ml (6 1/3 tbsp)	Milk

Preheat oven to 218°C (425°F).

Sift the dry ingredients together. Cut the fat into the flour with the aid of a pastry blender. Cut until the pieces are the size of uncooked rice grains. Make a well in the center of the mixture and add all of the milk at once. Using a 4-tined fork, cut through with 25 strokes to make the dough form a ball. Place on a very lightly floured bread board. Knead lightly 10 times with the fingertips. Roll out the dough, using 1/2″ thick parallel guides to achieve the desired uniform thickness. Cut with a biscuit cutter as efficiently as possible without cutting into the next biscuit. Use a spatula to transfer the biscuits to a baking sheet, leaving about 1/2″ between biscuits. Re-roll the remaining dough scraps. Keep these biscuits separate from the first ones, but place them on the same baking sheet. Bake at 218°C (425°F) until a pleasing golden brown (~ 12 to 15 minutes).

PROCEDURE

6. **Baking conditions for biscuits**—Prepare the basic formula and bake according to the following directions. The re-worked and re-rolled biscuits can be baked on the same sheet, but keep them separate so that first-rolling products can be judged against other first-rolling products, and so that judging can be done similarly on the re-rolled ones.

    a. *No preheating*—Prepare the basic formula, but place in a cold oven. Immediately set the oven at 218°C (425°F) and continue baking according to the basic formula.

    b. *Preheated oven, 150°C (300°F)*—Prepare the basic formula, but bake at 150°C (300°F). Note the baking time.

    c. *Preheated oven, 204°C (400°F)*—Prepare the basic formula, but bake at 204° (400°F). Note the baking time.

    d. *Preheated oven, 218°C (425°F)*—Prepare the basic formula. Note the baking time.

    e. *Preheated oven, 232°C (450°F)*—Prepare the basic formula, but bake at 232°C (450°F). Note the baking time.

    f. *30 minutes bench time*—Prepare the basic formula, but let the cut biscuits sit on the bench for 30 minutes before baking in a preheated oven at 218°C (425°F).

7. **Variations in types and amounts of leavening agents**—Prepare the basic formula for each of the following variations, noting carefully the

variations required in the ingredients. Bake according to the basic formula directions.

a. *Tartrate baking powder*—Prepare the basic formula, but use 7.2 g tartrate baking powder to replace the double-acting baking powder.

b. *2 times tartrate baking powder*—Prepare the basic formula, but use 14.4 g tartrate baking powder in place of the double-acting baking powder.

c. *3 times tartrate baking powder*—Prepare the basic formula, but use 21.6 g tartrate baking powder in place of the double-acting baking powder.

d. *2 times double-acting baking powder*—Prepare the basic formula, but use 14.4 g double-acting baking powder.

e. *3 times double-acting baking powder*—Prepare the basic formula, but use 21.6 g double-acting baking powder.

f. *Sour milk and soda*—Prepare the basic formula, but substitute 104 ml sour milk (made by mixing 7 ml lemon juice and 97 ml milk and letting it stand for 10 minutes) for the milk in the basic formula. Also, omit the baking powder and add 2 g soda.

EVALUATION

With a ruler, measure the height of the baked biscuits. Compare the percent increase of the various modifications being tested. If the biscuits have noticeably different heights at different points on the surface, measure the highest and lowest points and use the mean of these two measurements as the height of the biscuit for calculations. Sensory evaluation should include an assessment of the appearance of the crust, including color and any distinguishing features such as baking powder spots. Interior evaluation should include crumb color, tenderness (as determined by the number of chews), moistness, and flavor. In evaluating flavor, be very careful to note the overtones of flavor that may be obvious when air is exhaled sharply after swallowing the sample.

STUDY QUESTIONS

1. Which of the leavening agents tested (air, steam, and chemical leaveners) apparently caused the least leavening to occur? On the basis of this experiment, is it appropriate to conclude that air is an unimportant leavening agent? Explain your answer.

2. Under what experimental conditions was the greatest amount of leavening generated by steam in popovers?

3. Did the conditions under which angel cakes were baked have very much influence on the volume of the baked cake? Why is this so?

CHART 8.3.4 CHEMICAL LEAVENING AGENTS—BISCUITS

Treatment	Volume		Crust		Interior			
	Final ht. (mm)	% increase*	Color	Appear-ance	Color	Tender-ness (# chews)	Moist-ness	Flavor
6. Baking condition								
a. No preheat, 218°C								
b. Preheat, 150°C								
c. Preheat, 204°C								
d. Preheat, 218°C (Control)								
e. Preheat, 232°C								
f. 30 min. bench								
7. Variations								
a. 1x tartrate								
b. 2x tartrate								
c. 3x tartrate								
1x double acting b.p. (control, see 6d)								
d. 2x double acting								
e. 3x double acting								
f. Sour milk + soda								

$$*\% \text{ increase} = \frac{\text{final height} - \text{original height}}{\text{original height}} \times 100$$

Name

ADDITIONAL OBSERVATIONS AND NOTES

4. On the basis of the popover experiment, is it helpful to preheat (a) the containers and/or (b) oven when making popovers?

5. When soda and an acid are used as leavening ingredients, is bench time important? What precautions should be considered when developing recipes containing these ingredients?

6. Is the color of gingerbread influenced by the pH of the batter? If so, how? Is volume related to the pH of the batter? If so, how?

7. Do baking conditions influence the final volume of biscuits leavened with a double-acting baking powder? Cite examples from this experiment to illustrate your answer.

8. What changes are evident in baking powder biscuits as the level of baking powder is increased? Which type of baking powder can be used at the higher level? What problems become evident when too much baking powder is used?

9. Is it possible to tell whether a biscuit is baked from an alkaline dough? If so, how?

9
Breads

The structural element that is essential in breads is a protein complex in wheat. This complex, gluten, is developed when wheat flour is moistened and manipulated, as occurs when making batters and doughs. The mixing period is the time when the proteins in wheat flour begin to associate and form what appear to be almost rubber-like strands if manipulated long enough. Manipulation of batters and doughs to achieve the appropriate extent of gluten development is essential to creating the desired structure of various baked products.

Gluten strands show remarkable extensibility during the early part of baking. Until the temperature of the mixture rises to the point where the proteins denature, these strands stretch to give increasingly larger volume to the overall product and to promote thinner, more tender cell walls at the same time. The ability of gases to expand with the intense heat of the oven and the stretchy character of gluten work synergistically to help in achieving baked products with good texture and volume. The final requisite for utilizing the unique qualities of gluten is denaturation before the strands are stretched to the breaking point and while the gases in the cells are still exerting sufficient pressure to maintain the extended volume of the product.

If gluten strands are stretched to the breaking point before denaturation occurs, the structure will collapse into a somewhat compact, gummy product of limited palatability. Another cause of fallen baked products can be reduced pressure in the cells if the oven door is opened: The air from the room cools the gases in the cells, causing the cells to collapse. The gluten is still present in the baked product, but the cells will form a compact mass rather than being stretched to yield a tender product with a large volume and a delicate cell structure.

The experiments in this chapter are designed to help reveal the remarkable characteristics of gluten and the importance of this protein complex in quick and yeast breads. Flour from other cereals does not possess this same structural quality despite the fact that other cereals also are sources of plant proteins. Rye is the only other cereal known to have even a small fraction of the structural qualities possessed by wheat gluten. Triticale, a hybrid of wheat and rye, can contribute some structure, too.

EXPERIMENT 9.1—WHEAT GLUTEN
OBJECTIVES

Upon completion of the experiment, you will be able to:

1. Characterize the development of wheat gluten in batters and doughs.
2. Compare the differences in behavior between the protein in all purpose, cake, pastry, bread, rye, and triticale flours.
3. Conceptualize the changes the gluten complex undergoes during the baking period, from the stretchable complex to the denatured primary structure of the baked product.
4. Describe the factors influencing gluten development in a variety of baked products.

BASIC FORMULA—GLUTEN BALL

110 g (1 c)	Flour
60 ml (1/4 c)	Water

Use a fork to stir the dough that forms as the water is added to the flour. Add only enough water to make a stiff dough. Use less than the amount indicated if the dough can be worked without adding all 60 ml. Add more than 60 ml if necessary to make the dough. Record the exact amount of water used. After the water is added, knead the dough vigorously for 5 minutes, but without adding more flour. Place the ball in a strong muslin cloth. Hold the wrapped ball under a slow stream of cold water and manipulate the ball to begin to wash the starch from the dough. If the water looks cloudy or milky, there is still starch in the ball. Patiently continue the process until the water runs clear as it drains from the cloth.

When the water begins to look clear, open the cloth and scrape the cream-colored scraps together. Also, gather together any cream-colored particles that may be in the sink or on the outside of the cloth. This cream-colored material looks insignificant, but it is the gluten. When the starch has been washed away completely, the gluten mass will be quite cohesive and worked into a ball. Additional washing can be done without the cloth to eliminate any pockets of white starch that may be visible as the gluten is manipulated. It is imperative that all the starch be removed because starch will interfere with optimal expansion of the gluten ball during baking.

Before baking the gluten balls prepared in the class, class members should manipulate the various types to experience their elasticity and cohesiveness. Then the balls should be weighed. After weighing, bake the balls on pieces of foil in ovens preheated to 232°C (450°F). After baking 15 minutes, turn the temperature to 150°C (300°F) and continue baking another 30 minutes without opening the oven door. Cool briefly before weighing and measuring the volume. Cut in half to reveal the interior structure.

PROCEDURE

1. **Type of flour**—Using the flour assigned, prepare 1 gluten ball, according to the basic formula.

   a. *All purpose flour*—Prepare the basic formula using all purpose flour. This flour will serve as the control against which the others will be assessed.

   b. *Cake flour*—Prepare the basic formula using cake flour.

   c. *Pastry flour*—Prepare the basic formula using pastry flour.

   d. *Bread flour*—Prepare the basic formula using bread flour.

   e. *Rye flour*—Prepare the basic formula using rye flour.

   f. *Rye flour and all purpose flour*—Prepare the basic formula, but use 55 g rye flour and 55 g all purpose flour.

   g. *Whole wheat flour*—Prepare the basic formula using whole wheat flour.

   h. *Oat blend flour*—Prepare the basic formula using oat blend flour.

   i. *Triticale flour*—Prepare the basic formula using triticale flour.

2. **Baking conditions**—Prepare the basic formula using all purpose flour.

   a. *Cold oven, 232°C (450°F)*—Place the gluten ball (all purpose flour) in a cold oven; immediately begin to heat the oven on a setting of 232°C (450°F). Note the time required to set the structure.

   b. *Preheated oven, 150°C (300°F)*—Bake the (all purpose flour) gluten ball in a preheated oven at 150°C (300°F) until the structure is set. Note the time required.

   c. *Preheated oven, 177°C (350°F)*—Bake the (all purpose flour) gluten ball at 177°C (350°F) until the structure is set. Note the time required.

   d. *Preheated oven, 204°C (400°F)*—Bake the (all purpose flour) gluten ball at 204°C (400°F) until the structure is set. Note the time required.

   e. *Preheated oven, 232°C (450°F), open door*—Bake the (all purpose flour) gluten ball in an oven (with a window) at 232°C. When the gluten ball is stretching actively and is enlarged significantly, open the oven door wide open for 30 seconds. Close the door and continue baking until the structure is set.

EVALUATION

Prior to baking   Two evaluations are done prior to baking. The first is handling as many of the different types of gluten balls as possible so that the differences in the character of the undenatured gluten from the various flours can be experienced. The second part of evaluation at this point is weighing the balls. This is done so that a comparison can be made between the initial weight of the flour and the significantly smaller weight of the gluten. Since flour contains a large proportion of starch, this difference is to be expected, but the weighing (despite its inaccuracies due to loss of gluten during the washing process and excess water clinging to the ball) does help to provide a realistic picture of the significant role that a relatively small amount of protein plays in baked products and their structure.

During baking   While the balls are baking, watch through oven windows to observe the behavior of the various treatments. Do not open the oven door during baking. Record the changes noted during baking.

After baking   Let the balls cool briefly after baking and then measure their volume. The volume is an indication of the strength of the gluten. Also weigh the balls. Then cut the balls in half to reveal the interior structure. Note the thickness of the cell walls and the size of the cells. Take hold of the strands in the center and note the relative strength in the various products. These balls are intended to illustrate the characteristics of gluten and are *not* considered to be a food. Sensory evaluation is done only by looking at the balls and touching them.

STUDY QUESTIONS

1. Compare the relative structural qualities of the various items tested. Compare the amount of protein in the various products.

2. What changes take place from the time wheat flour is first moistened until a gluten ball has been baked?

3. What can be done to improve the structural characteristics of baked products that are likely to fall?

CHART 9.1   GLUTEN STRUCTURE—BEFORE AND AFTER BAKING GLUTEN BALLS

Treatment	Weight		Character-istics of raw ball	Volume baked ball (ml)	Descrip-tion of	Interior		
	Prior to baking (g)	After baking (g)				Texture of cell exterior	Cell walls	Strand strength
1. Type of flour a. All purpose (Control)								
b. Cake								
c. Pastry								
d. Bread								
e. Rye								
f. Rye + all purpose								
g. Whole wheat								
h. Oat								
i. Triticale								
2. Baking conditions a. No preheat, 232°C								
b. Preheat, 150°C								
c. Preheat, 177°C								
d. Preheat, 204°C								
e. Preheat, 232°C; open door 30 sec								

Name

ADDITIONAL OBSERVATIONS AND NOTES

EXPERIMENT 9.2—YEAST BREADS
OBJECTIVES

Upon completion of the experiment, you will be able to:

1. Explain the procedure for making yeast doughs, outline the precautions that need to be observed, and assess the quality of yeast products.
2. Identify the practical use of various types of flour in yeast products.
3. Discuss the importance of kneading and of control of water (or other liquid) to flour ratios in bread dough.

BASIC FORMULA—BREAD

7 g (1 pkg)	Yeast, dry
118 ml (1/2 c)	Water at 35°C
4 g (1 tsp)	Shortening
6 g (1 1/2 tsp)	Sugar
3 g (1/2 tsp)	Salt
200 g (1 7/8 c)	All purpose flour

Add yeast to 59 ml water after being certain that the water temperature is 35°C (95°F). Barely melt the shortening. Place sugar, salt, and remaining 59 ml water in a mixing bowl and add the shortening and then the yeast-water mixture. Stir to blend. Gradually begin adding the flour while mixing slowly with an electric mixer.

Add just enough flour to make a very soft paste. Beat with the electric mixer until smooth. Remove beater blades and scrape them thoroughly with a rubber spatula to avoid losing any dough. Continue mixing by hand with a wooden spoon while adding just enough flour to make a smooth, non-sticky, rather soft dough. If all of the weighed flour is used, weigh another 25 g and use what is needed to make the dough manageable. Knead the dough on a bread board by folding the far edge of the dough to meet the front edge and pushing firmly with the heel of both hands before rotating the dough 90° and repeating the process until 100 kneading strokes have been completed. Very lightly coat dough with oil. Place in a beaker large enough to allow the dough to double in size and cover with aluminum foil.

Let rise 30 minutes in a water bath maintained at 32°C (90°F). Punch dough down after estimating the volume of the risen dough. Shape into a loaf and place in a greased loaf pan 5 3/4" × 3 1/2" × 2". Return to the water bath and let rise until double in volume. Meanwhile preheat the oven to 220°C (425°F). Bake for about 15 minutes (until bread sounds hollow when tapped). Remove from pan immediately and cool on a wire rack.

PROCEDURE

1. Amount of kneading

   a. *No kneading*—Prepare the basic formula, but do not knead the dough at all. Simply prepare it for rising and proceed according to the basic formula.

    b. *50 strokes kneading*—Prepare the basic formula, but knead the dough only 50 times. Proceed according to the basic formula.

    c. *100 strokes (control)*—Prepare the basic formula. This is the control loaf for judging all of the variations.

    d. *200 strokes kneading*—Prepare the basic formula, but knead the dough 200 times. Be sure to maintain the same kneading technique and pressure throughout the process.

    e. *500 strokes kneading*—Prepare the basic formula, but knead 500 times using exactly the same technique and pressure throughout the kneading process.

2. **Amount of flour**

    a. *Too little flour*—Prepare the basic formula, but reduce the weight of flour to 160 g. If the dough is too soft to knead, simply knead it in the bowl with a spoon. Proceed with the rising according to the basic formula.

    b. *Excess flour*—Prepare the basic formula, but have a weighed amount of flour available during the kneading process. Work as much of this flour as possible into the dough during the kneading process. This is done by generously and frequently adding flour to the board. Weigh the flour remaining after kneading to determine the total amount of flour in the dough. Note how the handling characteristics changed during kneading as more flour was worked in.

3. **Type of liquid**

    a. *Milk*—Prepare the basic formula, using milk in place of the water.

4. **Type of flour**—The ratios of different flours used are based on the weight of the individual products, as indicated in the directions below.

    a. *Whole wheat flour, 25%*—Prepare the basic formula, but use 50 g of whole wheat flour and 150 g of all purpose flour.

    b. *Whole wheat flour, 50%*—Prepare the basic formula, but use 100 g of whole wheat flour and 100 g of all purpose flour.

    c. *Whole wheat flour, 100%*—Prepare the basic formula, but use 200 g of whole wheat flour and no all purpose flour. If it is necessary to add flour during kneading, use only whole wheat flour.

    d. *Soy flour, 25%*—Prepare the basic formula, but use 50 g of soy flour and 150 g of all purpose flour.

    e. *Soy flour, 50%*—Prepare the basic formula, but use 100 g of soy flour and 100 g of all purpose flour.

    f. *Rye flour*—Prepare the basic formula, but use 50 g of rye flour and 150 g of all purpose flour.

    g. *Rye flour, 50%*—Prepare the basic formula, but use 100 g of rye flour and 100 g of all purpose flour.

h. *25% rye flour, 25% whole wheat flour, 25% soy flour, and 25% all purpose flour*—Prepare the basic formula, but use 50 g each of rye flour, whole wheat flour, soy flour, and all purpose flour.

i. *Triticale flour, 50%*—Prepare the basic formula, but use 100 g of triticale flour and 100 g of all purpose flour.

EVALUATION

Objective testing   The loaves should be removed from the pans when the bread is removed from the oven and then cooled on wire racks. Volume of all of the loaves should be measured, preferably by using the volumeter. Then cut the loaf in half and remove a slice about 1/2″ thick and make a copy using a copy machine, digital camera, or ink print. The copy provides a record of the uniformity of texture and evidence of the thickness of cell walls.

Subjective testing   Subjective testing is done to assess the curvature and texture of the crust, as well as its color. The interior should have slightly coarse, even cells with uniformly medium-thick cell walls, and the color should be uniform throughout. Tenderness can be assessed by counting the number of chews. Any tendency toward crumbliness also should be noted, because a crumbly texture is inconsistent with the requirement that a bread be able to serve as a base for spreads and sandwich fillings. Flavor also should be noted.

STUDY QUESTIONS

1. Outline the basic procedure for making yeast breads. What temperature range is safe for rehydrating yeast? At what temperature should fermentation take place?

2. What is the effect of increasing the amount of flour in a bread dough? Why does this occur?

3. What is the result of using milk rather than water as the liquid for making bread? Is milk a suitable liquid to use in making breads? Why?

4. Is kneading beneficial to the quality of bread? What effect does kneading have on bread? Is it possible to knead bread dough too much? Too little? Describe the finished product that results when bread dough is kneaded (a) too little and (b) too much. Why do these results occur?

5. Is it possible to substitute soy flour for all purpose flour in breads? If so, up to approximately what level? What might be a motivation for making this substitution?

6. What is the result of trying to make a bread with a high percentage of rye flour? What modifications can be made to achieve an acceptable product?

7. Compare the characteristics of breads made using (a) 50% soy, (b) 50% rye, and (c) 50% triticale.

8. What might be a motivating reason for developing a bread made with a mixture of different flours? How successful were the different blends that were illustrated in this experiment? What avenues were suggested for further research?

9. Can whole wheat and all purpose flours be used interchangeably in a bread recipe? Explain your answer.

CHART 9.2 ASSESSMENT OF THE VALUE OF KNEADING AND THE POTENTIAL FOR MAKING SUBSTITUTIONS IN BREAD RECIPES

Treatment	Volume (ml)	Crust		Interior cells		Interior color	Tender-ness (# chews)	Flavor
		Color	Texture	Uniformity	Cell size			
1. Kneading a. None								
b. 50x								
c. 100x								
d. 200x								
e. 500x								
2. Amount flour a. Little								
b. Excess (____ g)								
3. Milk								
4. Type of flour a. 25% whole wheat								
b. 50% whole wheat								
c. 100% whole wheat								
d. 25% soy								
e. 50% soy								
f. 25% rye								
g. 50% rye								
h. 25% rye, 25% soy, 25% whole wheat, 25% all purpose								
i. 50% triticale								

Name

ADDITIONAL OBSERVATIONS AND NOTES

EXPERIMENT 9.3—FACTORS INFLUENCING MUFFINS
OBJECTIVES

Upon completion of the experiment, you will be able to:

1. Evaluate quality in muffins and theorize as to the reasons for possible variations from the accepted standard.
2. Explain the role of each of the following in muffin recipes: sugar, egg, milk, flour, and fat.
3. Predict, based on theory, the effect of modifying the levels of any of the ingredients in a standard muffin formula.
4. Explain the development of gluten in muffins and identify the extent of development by evaluating a baked muffin.

BASIC FORMULA—MUFFINS

24 g (1/2)	Egg
118 ml (1/2 c)	Milk
12 g (1 tbsp)	Salad oil
110 g (1 c)	All purpose flour
12.5 g (1 tbsp)	Sugar
5.5 g (1 1/2 tbsp)	Baking powder, double acting
1.5 g (1/4 tsp)	Salt

Beat the egg until blended, but not foamy. Add the milk and salad oil; then beat gently with an eggbeater just enough to blend the liquids homogeneously. Sift the dry ingredients together in a mixing bowl. Make a well in the dry ingredients and add the liquid mixture all at once. Stir gently, but efficiently, with a wooden spoon. Count each stroke. Try to have all of the dry ingredients moistened and stirred in with 15 strokes. If some dry flour remains, continue mixing just until no dry flour is left. Be sure to count the total number of strokes used.

Lightly grease the bottom of 4 cups in a muffin pan. Balance the muffin pan. Weigh 55 g of batter into the first greased compartment. If possible, do this by pushing batter from a large spoon into the cup without having to get more batter from the bowl. Without doing more mixing, proceed to weigh out (in the remaining 3 greased compartments) 3 more muffins, each weighing 55 g. Identify the sequence in which the muffins are placed.

Bake in a preheated oven at 218°C (425°F) oven for 20 minutes or until golden brown. Remove muffins from the pan immediately and cool on a wire rack for evaluation.

PROCEDURE

1. **Amount of mixing**—For this series, follow the basic formula, but use the exact number of strokes indicated for each variation. Be very careful to avoid manipulating the batter as each muffin is scooped from the mixing bowl and into the baking pan.

a. *5 strokes*—Mix the batter only 5 strokes. Be sure to dish a representative portion of the dry as well as of the liquid ingredients into the muffin pan.

b. *15 strokes or until just blended*—Prepare the basic formula. This batch will serve as the control for comparison of the variations in this entire experiment. The batter should be lumpy, but with no dry flour remaining.

c. *35 strokes*—Prepare the basic formula, but mix the liquid and dry ingredients together a total of 35 strokes.

d. *100 strokes*—Prepare the basic formula, but mix the liquid and dry ingredients a total of 100 strokes. Record the appearance of the batter when 5 strokes have been used to blend. Again, record the appearance of the batter at 15, 35, and 100 strokes. The description of the changes in the batter at various stages of mixing is a part of the report to the class members who were not able to see the batter progress.

2. **Amount of sugar**—Note carefully the number of strokes required to mix the batter to the desired end point. Record the length of time required for achieving the golden brown color during baking.

   a. *No sugar*—Prepare the basic formula, but omit the sugar.

   b. *6 g sugar*—Prepare the basic formula, but use only 6 g (1/2x) sugar.

   c. *25 g sugar*—Prepare the basic formula, but use 25 g (2x) sugar.

3. **Amount and kind of egg protein**—Count the number of strokes required for mixing. Carefully note the baking time required to achieve the desired degree of browning.

   a. *No egg*—Prepare the basic formula, but omit the egg.

   b. *Egg white only*—Prepare the basic formula, but use 24 g of egg white and no egg yolk.

   c. *Egg yolk only*—Prepare the basic formula, but use 24 g of egg yolk and no egg white.

   d. *48 g whole egg (2x)*—Prepare the basic formula, but double the amount of egg (total of 48 g whole egg).

   e. *Egg substitute*—Prepare the basic formula, but use 24 g of an egg substitute in place of the egg.

4. **Kinds of milk**—Observe the batter during mixing for any noticeable differences in mixing characteristics. Watch the baking to see whether differences in browning are noted.

   a. *Fat free milk*—Prepare the basic formula, but use fat free milk (118 ml) in place of whole milk.

   b. *Half and half*—Prepare the basic formula, but use half and half in place of whole milk.

   c. *Soy milk*—Prepare the basic formula, but use soy milk in place of whole milk.

d. *Evaporated milk*—Prepare the basic formula, but use undiluted evaporated milk in place of whole milk.

5. **Type and amount of fat**—This series is designed to demonstrate the effect of substituting various fats in place of oil. These variations are to be compared with the control (sample 1b). In addition, this series uses margarine as the fat to demonstrate the effect of modifying the amount of fat.

   a. *Benecol®*—Prepare the basic formula, but use melted Benecol® in place of the salad oil.

   b. *Butter*—Prepare the basic formula, but use melted butter in place of the salad oil.

   c. *Margarine*—Prepare the basic formula, but use melted margarine in place of the salad oil.

   d. *Double the fat*—Prepare the basic formula, but use 24 g of melted margarine in place of the salad oil.

   e. *No fat*—Prepare the basic formula, but use no fat.

6. **Type of flour**—These variations illustrate the role of gluten in muffins. If mixing has to be modified, be sure to count the number of strokes.

   a. *Cake flour*—Prepare the basic formula, but use 96 g (1 c) cake flour in place of all purpose flour.

   b. *Soy, whole wheat, and all purpose flour*—Prepare the basic formula, but use 27.5 g soy flour, 27.5 g whole wheat flour, and 55 g all purpose flour (25%, 25%, 50%, respectively).

7. **Microwave cookery**

   a. *Microwave*—Prepare the basic formula, but bake in the microwave oven. Be sure to use 4 custard cups with paper linings for this variation. Microwave for 2 minutes.

EVALUATION

Preparation of batter   Descriptions of batter appearance and the number of strokes used for the various batches are important information. These should be recorded and referred to when conducting a sensory evaluation of the baked muffins.

Objective evaluation   Volume is a very useful measure when evaluating muffins. Since all muffins were baked with the same amount of batter, the volume of only 1 muffin from each batch needs to be measured. Then cut it in half vertically and place on display to provide a muffin for visual evaluation and for making an ink print or photocopy. Use the other 3 for sensory evaluation.

Sensory evaluation   Much can be determined about muffin quality simply by looking at them. Begin by noting the silhouette of the muffin. Note particularly the shape or conformation of the top crust. Examine the texture as well as the general outline. High quality muffins have a gently rounded (not a flat nor peaked) top, and the crust has soft undulations resembling the texture of a head of cauliflower. The color should be a golden brown. Exterior evaluation is important to help distinguish subtle differences produced by the different variations in this experiment. Interior evaluation also needs to be done carefully, beginning with cell structure. Note the appearance of the cell walls. Look for any suggestion of a waxy character. Note also the crumb color. Uniformity of cells also is important. A muffin of high quality will have relatively uniform, somewhat coarse cells, but will not show evidence of tunnels. Tunnels, large breaks in the cell structure usually directed toward the highest point in the muffin, are considered undesirable. Flavor should be evaluated for initial reaction and for aftertaste experienced when breath is exhaled sharply after swallowing. Tenderness is judged by counting the number of chews.

STUDY QUESTIONS

1. What is the role of each of the following ingredients in muffins: flour, milk, egg, sugar, baking powder, salt, and fat?

2. What is the result of modifying the type and/or the amount of all purpose flour in a muffin formula?

3. Can different forms of eggs be substituted in muffins? Describe the effect of using the various forms and also of omitting egg in a muffin formula.

4. What effect(s) on muffins can be noted when sugar is (a) decreased or omitted and (b) increased in muffins?

5. Compare the ease of substituting fats in a muffin recipe with similar substitutions in pastry. Explain the rationale for your answer.

6. Describe a well prepared muffin. How does the amount of mixing influence the likelihood of a muffin receiving a high score?

7. What effects could be observed when various milks are substituted in a muffin formula? Which, if any, cannot be used satisfactorily?

8. How did the muffins baked in the microwave oven compare with those baked in a conventional oven?

9. Did variations in any of the ingredients require a change in the amount of mixing? If so, which variation(s)?

CHART 9.3.1   EFFECTS OF VARIATIONS ON MUFFIN BATTERS

Treatment	# mixing strokes required	Baking time	Description of batter after mixing
1. Mixing a. 5 strokes	XXX		
b. 15 strokes (control)	XXX		
c. 35 strokes	XXX		
d. 100 strokes	XXX		
2. Amount of sugar a. None			XXX
b. 6 g			XXX
12.5 g (See 1.b)			XXX
c. 25 g			XXX
3. Amount and kind of egg a. No egg			XXX
b. White only			XXX
c. Yolk only			XXX
d. 2x egg			XXX
e. Substitute (_____ used)			XXX
4. Kinds of milk a. Fat free			
Whole (See 1.b)			
b. Half and half			
c. Soy milk			
d. Evaporated (undiluted)			
5. Type and amount of fat a. Benecol®			XXX
b. Butter			XXX
c. Margarine			XXX
d. 2x margarine			XXX
e. No fat			XXX
6. Type of flour a. Cake flour			
All purpose (See 1.b)			
b. 25% soy, 25% whole wheat, 50% all purpose			
7. Microwave oven a. 2 min.			XXX

Name

ADDITIONAL OBSERVATIONS AND NOTES

CHART 9.3.2   EVALUATION OF MUFFINS

Treatment	Vol.* (ml)	Exterior appearance	Interior		Color	Flavor	Tender-ness (# chews)	Overall rating
			Texture					
			Cell size, walls	Uniform-ity, tunnels				
1. Mixing								
a. 5x								
b. 15x (Control)								
c. 35x								
d. 100x								
2. Sugar								
a. None								
b. 6 g								
c. 25 g								
3. Egg								
a. None								
b. White								
c. Yolk								
d. 2x								
e. Substitute								
4. Milk								
a. Fat free								
b. Half and half								
c. Soy milk								
d. Evaporated								
5. Fat								
a. Benecol®								
b. Butter								
c. Margarine								
d. 2x margarine								
e. None								
6. Flour								
a. Cake								
b. Soy, whole wheat, all purpose								
7. Microwave								

*Determine with volumeter or calculate the mean height by measuring at the muffin edge and at the highest point. Use this mean height to calculate the volume.

Name

ADDITIONAL OBSERVATIONS AND NOTES

EXPERIMENT 9.4—CHARACTERISTICS OF BISCUITS
OBJECTIVES

Upon completion of the experiment, you will be able to:

1. Explain the effect of manipulation on gluten development in biscuit dough.
2. Interpret the effect of varying the methods of incorporating the fat and of varying the type of fat in biscuits.
3. Discuss the effect of varying the ratio of milk to flour in biscuits.
4. Evaluate biscuits according to accepted criteria and diagnose probable errors in making biscuits failing to meet these standards.
5. Assess the use of a microwave oven as a means of baking biscuits.

BASIC FORMULA—BISCUITS

116 g (1 c)	All purpose flour
5.4 g (1 1/2 tsp)	Baking powder, double-acting
1.5 g (1/4 tsp)	Salt
24 g (2 tbsp)	Shortening
95 ml (6 1/3 tbsp)	Milk

Sift the dry ingredients together. Cut the fat into the flour using a pastry blender until the pieces are the size of uncooked rice grains. Make a well in this mixture, and add all of the milk at once. With a 4-tined fork, cut through the ingredients and form a dough ball using only 25 strokes. Place the dough ball on a breadboard that has been floured very lightly. Knead lightly 10 times using the fingertips. Roll out the dough, using 1/2"-thick parallel guides to make the dough a uniform thickness. Cut with a biscuit cutter. Avoid cutting into the next biscuit, but cut as efficiently as possible. With a spatula, transfer the biscuits to a baking sheet, leaving about 1/2" between biscuits. Re-roll the remaining dough and cut biscuits. Place on same baking sheet, but separated from the biscuits from the first rolling. Bake at 218°C (425°F) until a pleasing golden brown (about 12–15 minutes).

PROCEDURE

1. **Amount of stirring**—Prepare the basic formula for each of the following variations. Be careful to cut the biscuits with vertical sides and transfer them carefully to the baking sheet to retain their shape.

    a. *Stir 15 times*—Prepare the basic formula, but stir only 15 times with a fork.

    b. *Stir 25 times (control)*—Prepare the basic formula.

    c. *Stir 50 times*—Prepare the basic formula, but stir a total of 50 times with the fork.

2. **Amount of kneading**—Prepare the basic formula for each of the following variations. Although different groups can be assigned the mixing and weighing, one student should do all of the kneading for the variations in procedure 2. This will eliminate the inevitable variations in kneading that would occur with more than one person performing this key step.

   a. *Knead 0 times*—Prepare the basic formula, but do not knead the dough at all. Simply press it into a mass on the board with essentially no manipulation of the dough.

   b. *Knead 10 times (control)*—Prepare the basic formula.

   c. *Knead 30 times*—Prepare the basic recipe but knead the dough 30 times, being sure to have the kneading done by the person who kneads procedure 2b.

3. **Amount and kind of milk**—Prepare the basic recipe for each of the variations below. Handle the dough carefully, trying to avoid varying the amount of manipulation even though the dough handles differently.

   a. *80 ml milk*—Prepare the basic formula, but use only 80 ml milk.

   b. *110 ml milk*—Prepare the basic formula, but use 110 ml milk.

   c. *95 ml soy milk*—Prepare the basic formula, but use 95 ml soy milk.

4. **Ways of incorporating fat**—Ordinarily shortening is cut into the flour and other dry ingredients until the pieces are about the size of uncooked rice grains. This series illustrates variations from this technique.

   a. *Very fine particles*—Prepare the basic formula, but cut the shortening into particles as fine as possible.

   b. *Melted, added with milk*—Prepare the basic formula, but melt the shortening, cool a little, and then add to the dry ingredients along with the milk.

5. **Type of fat**—Prepare the basic formula for these variations, but substitute the type of fat indicated below.

   a. *Butter*—Prepare the basic formula, but use 28 g (2 tbsp) butter in place of the shortening. Note that this weight represents an equal volume of fat, but is slightly heavier than the fat in the basic formula because of the water content of butter.

   b. *Margarine*—Prepare the basic formula, but substitute 28 g margarine for the shortening. As was true with the butter substitution in procedure 5a, this is an equal substitution based on fat content.

   c. *Benecol®*—Prepare the basic formula, but substitute 28 g Benecol® for the shortening. This weight will replace an equal volume of shortening.

   d. *Salad oil*—Prepare the basic formula, but substitute 29.5 ml salad oil for the shortening. The salad oil should be stirred into the milk and added all at once, as described in the basic formula. Note that the fat is not cut in.

6. **Microwave oven**—Prepare the basic formula, but place the biscuits on a flat non-metallic dish. Bake according to the directions given for the microwave oven being used. If no directions are available, microwave for 1 minute 30 seconds, or until biscuits are firm and not doughy. Let stand at least 2 minutes before evaluating.

EVALUATION

Objective evaluation   With a ruler, measure the height of all of the biscuits in the batch. For those with slanting tops, measure the highest point and the lowest point and determine the mean value. Determine the mean height for the entire batch. If time allows, measure the volume of 2 of the biscuits from the first rolling in the volumeter.

Subjective evaluation   Evaluate the exterior of the biscuit by first looking critically at the upper surface of the biscuit. Note whether it is parallel with the plate and whether the surface is flat. Also observe any brown spots that may be present. Next, note the appearance of the sides, looking specifically at whether there is evidence of cracking or layering. On the bottom, check to see whether the edges are curling.

Interior evaluation should be directed toward noting flakiness. This can be judged after breaking the biscuit in half horizontally and then rubbing the interior surface lightly with a finger. If the biscuit rolls up in layers, it is said to be flaky. Color and flavor should be noted. Tenderness is an important measure and can be done by counting the number of chews. Be sure to decide what portion of the biscuit (interior only or some exterior surface, too) individual judges are to use when counting the number of chews.

Criteria for the exterior of a high quality biscuit include straight sides, flat upper and lower surfaces with no bending toward the edges, and a pleasing golden-brown color (with or without flecks of brown). A flaky interior with a white color, blended flavor with no aftertaste, and a tender crumb are other desirable characteristics. The sides of the biscuit will crack in layers a bit when the biscuit is made correctly. This cracking is evidence of flakiness and is not a negative point in evaluation. Of course, the volume should be good, and the interior should not seem doughy.

STUDY QUESTIONS

1. In making biscuits, what is the optimum amount of (a) stirring, (b) kneading? What is the result of too little (a) stirring, (b) kneading? Compare the kneading technique for making biscuits with the technique for yeast bread and explain why each is used.

2. What effect does over-kneading have on tenderness and volume of biscuits? Does over-stirring have the same result as over-kneading?

3. Why are biscuits kneaded?

4. Does the size of fat particles in biscuits have any effect on the finished product? Does melted fat give the same result as using solid shortening?

5. Highlight the differences that can be noted between biscuits made with the different fats used in this experiment.

6. What is the result of varying the level of milk in biscuits? Of using soy milk?

7. Can biscuits be baked satisfactorily in a microwave oven?

8. Select a biscuit that is not equal to the criteria for excellence described above. Identify what changes would need to be made in its preparation or formula in order to produce a biscuit of high quality.

CHART 9.4 EVALUATION OF BISCUITS

Treatment	Mean ht. (mm)	Vol./ 2 bis. (ml)	Exterior		Interior			
			Surfaces	Sides	Color	Flakiness	Tenderness (# chews)	Flavor
1. Stirring a. 15 x								
b. 25 x (control)								
c. 50 x								
2. Kneading a. None								
b. 10x (see 1b)								
c. 30x								
3. Milk a. 80 ml								
95 ml (see 1b)								
b. 110 ml								
c. 95 ml soy milk								
4. Incorp. fat a. Very fine								
Coarse (see 1b)								
b. Melted								
5. Type of fat a. Butter								
b. Margarine								
c. Benecol®								
d. Oil								
6. Microwave								

Name

ADDITIONAL OBSERVATIONS AND NOTES

EXPERIMENT 9.5—FACTORS INFLUENCING PANCAKES
OBJECTIVES

Upon completion of the experiment, you will be able to:

1. Identify the role of each of the ingredients in a basic pancake recipe.
2. Discuss the significance of temperature control when baking pancakes.
3. Evaluate pancakes according to established criteria and recommend appropriate changes in recipe or procedure for products deviating from the standard.
4. Explain the changes that result when variations are made in the levels of fat, sugar, eggs, and liquid, as well as when some ingredients are substituted (soy flour, sugar substitute, and egg substitute).
5. Assess the feasibility of baking pancakes in the microwave oven.

BASIC FORMULA—PANCAKES

70 g (10 tbsp)	All purpose flour
4 g (1 tsp)	Sugar
1.5 g (1/4 tsp)	Salt
5.4 g (1 1/2 tsp)	Baking powder
24 g (1/2)	Egg
118 ml (1/2 c)	Milk
15 ml (1 tbsp)	Salad oil

Sift the flour, sugar, salt, and baking powder together. In a separate bowl, beat the egg, and then beat in the milk and salad oil. Pour all of the liquid ingredients into the dry ingredients. Stir 50 strokes with a wooden spoon. If the batter is not smooth, continue stirring until it is smooth, being sure to record the total number of strokes used.

Preheat the griddle on a thermostatic unit (350°F) until cold water dropped on the skillet jumps around, but does not sizzle. Pour 40 ml batter on the skillet or griddle. Let bake on the first side until the bubbles that form and rise to the top of the pancake have popped and the bottom of the pancake is a pleasing, golden brown. Flip the pancake and brown the second side to a golden brown. Maintain the baking temperature throughout the baking period. Bake the remainder of the batter in 40 ml pancakes.

PROCEDURE

1. **Amount of fat**—For the variations in this series, follow the procedure for the basic formula, varying only the amount of shortening as indicated.

   a. *No fat*—Prepare the basic formula, but do not use any fat or oil.

   b. *15 ml oil (control)*—Prepare the basic formula. This is the control.

c. *30 ml oil*—Prepare the basic formula, but use a total of 30 ml oil (double the control amount).

2. **Amount of milk**—Use whole milk for all variations. Try to mix the same number of strokes indicated in the basic formula.

a. *90 ml milk*—Prepare the basic formula, but use only 90 ml milk.

b. *150 ml milk*—Prepare the basic formula, but use 150 ml milk.

3. **Amount and kind of sugar**—This series illustrates the effect of modifying the amount of sugar and also tests the use of a sugar substitute.

a. *No sugar*—Prepare the basic formula, but omit the sugar.

b. *8 g sugar*—Prepare the basic formula, but use 8 g (double the basic amount) of sugar.

c. *0.4 g sugar substitute*—Prepare the basic formula, but omit the sugar and use a sugar substitute.

4. **Baking temperature**—The basic formula is used, but the temperature of the griddle or skillet is varied according to the directions below. Be sure the skillet is at the temperature indicated before beginning baking. Test a few drops of water on the skillet or griddle when it reaches the test temperature. Describe the behavior of the water at the test temperature.

a. *150°C (300°F)*—Prepare the basic formula. Bake according to the directions in the basic formula, except bake at 150°C (300°F).

b. *204°C (400°F)*—Prepare the basic formula. Bake according to the directions in the basic formula, except bake at 204°C (400°F).

c. *Microwave oven*—Prepare the basic formula, but bake 15 seconds in the microwave oven. If desired, each pancake can be baked 5 seconds longer than the preceding one. Be sure to label the samples with the number of seconds each was baked.

5. **Flour substitutions**—Soy flour at 2 different levels and cake flour are substituted for part of the flour in these variations.

a. *17.5 g soy flour (25% of flour)*—Prepare the basic formula, but substitute part of the flour by using 17.5 g soy flour and 52.5 g all purpose flour. Be sure to mix the two flours together thoroughly before adding the liquid ingredients.

b. *35 g soy flour (50% of flour)*—Prepare the basic formula, but substitute part of the flour by using 35 g soy flour and 35 g all purpose flour. Be sure to mix the two flours together thoroughly before adding the liquid ingredients.

c. *Cake flour*—Prepare the basic formula, but substitute 60 g of cake flour for the all purpose flour. This amount gives an equal substitution by volume.

d. *Flax seed*—Prepare the basic formula, but add 40 g coarse, ground flax seed.

6. **Egg variations**—The following series illustrates various uses of egg and egg substitutes.

   a. *Egg substitute*—Prepare the basic formula, but use 24 g of liquid egg substitute for the egg.

   b. *Egg white as foam*—Prepare the basic formula, but use 8 g of yolk and 16 g of white in place of a whole egg. Include 8 g of yolk as described in the basic formula. Proceed to stir the batter as described in the basic formula. Beat the 16 g of egg white until the peaks just bend over. Quickly stir the foam into the batter and bake as described in the basic formula.

   c. *48 g egg (2x)*—Prepare the basic formula, but increase the egg to 48 g.

7. **Mixing**—Prepare the basic formula, but double the amount of stirring, making a total of 100 strokes.

EVALUATION

Objective evaluation Evaluate the volume of the pancakes by cutting one pancake in half and stacking the two halves with the cut sides on the same side. Place a ruler vertically against the cut edge and measure the height of the two stacked halves. Measure the diameter.

Subjective evaluation Evaluate the exterior by observing the attractiveness of the browning on the surface browned initially (served as the top side on the plate). The pancake also should be evaluated for tenderness (counting the number of chews), for texture (uniformity and actual size of cells), and flavor. To evaluate flavor, exhale sharply after swallowing to detect any aftertaste.

STUDY QUESTIONS

1. Does the level of fat have an influence on tenderness, volume, or diameter of the pancakes? If so, explain the specific effect(s).

2. What is the effect of decreasing the liquid in pancakes? Of increasing the liquid?

3. Does the change in the amount of sugar influence the finished product in an observable way? Explain your answer.

4. Describe the pancakes made with sugar substitute, and explain why they differ from those made with sugar.

5. What effect(s) can be noted, both subjectively and objectively, as a result of modifying baking temperatures? What temperature seems to

be optimum? Describe the appearance of the water test at the different temperatures used in the experiment.

6. Describe the pancakes made with (a) two levels of soy flour, (b) cake flour, and (c) flax seed. Are these substitutions satisfactory for making a quality product? If not, why not?

CHART 9.5   EVALUATION OF PANCAKES

Treatment	Ht. (mm)	Diameter (mm)	Appearance	Tenderness (# chews)	Texture		Flavor
					Cell size	Uniformity	
1. Fat a. None							
b. 15 ml (control)							
c. 30 ml							
2. Milk a. 90 ml							
118 ml (control) (see 1b)							
b. 150 ml							
3. Sugar a. None							
b. 8 g (2x)							
c. Substitute							
4. Temperature a. 150°C							
175°C (control) (see 1b)							
b. 204°C							
c. Microwave							
5. Flour sub. a. 25% soy							
b. 50% soy							
c. Cake							
d. Flax seed							
6. Egg a. Substitute							
b. White foam							
c. 48 g (2x)							
7. Mixing, 100 strokes							

Name

ADDITIONAL OBSERVATIONS AND NOTES

10
Shortened Cakes

Cakes, because of their somewhat richer formulas, require more mixing than quick breads to develop the gluten. Their complex ingredients afford the opportunity for variations in methods of mixing. The structure of shortened cakes is finer and the crumb is more tender than in breads. The delicacy of the structure makes shortened cakes susceptible to falling if their ratio of sugar to flour is elevated excessively or if gluten development or baking conditions are not optimal. The experiments in this chapter are designed to demonstrate the effects of variations in mixing methods and in levels of ingredients.

EXPERIMENT 10.1—METHODS OF MIXING SHORTENED CAKES
OBJECTIVES

Upon completion of the experiment, you will be able to:

1. Outline the basic procedures involved in making shortened cakes using the following methods: conventional, conventional meringue, conventional sponge, muffin, muffin-meringue, single-stage, pastry-blend, and solution.
2. Identify the advantages and disadvantages of each of the methods in Objective 1.
3. Evaluate shortened cakes on the basis of established criteria.

BASIC FORMULA—SHORTENED CAKE

56 g (1/4 c)	Butter
150 g (3/4 c)	Sugar
3 ml (1/2 tsp)	Vanilla
48 g (1)	Egg, beaten
150 g (1 1/2 c)	Cake flour
5.4 g (1 1/2 tsp)	Baking powder
2 g (1/4 tsp)	Salt
120 ml (1/2 c)	Milk

Line bottom of 2 cake pans (5 3/4″ × 3 1/2″ × 2″) with wax paper that is cut to fit the bottom without going up the sides. Preheat oven to 185°C (365°F).

Cream the butter, sugar, and vanilla together for 2 minutes on an electric mixer set at the speed indicated for creaming (use medium high if no creaming speed is shown). Pour the egg into the creamed mixture, and beat until light and somewhat fluffy. Remove from the mixer; scrape the beater blades with a rubber spatula. Add approximately one-third of the sifted mixture (flour, baking powder, and salt). With a wooden spoon, blend in the mixture using 50 strokes. Add half the milk, and stir 25 strokes. Then add the second third of the flour mixture and stir 50 more strokes. Add the last half of the milk; stir 25 strokes. Finally, add the last third of the flour mixture and stir 75 strokes (making a grand total of 225 strokes).

Pour 225 g of the batter into one cake pan and 225 g of batter into the second pan. Note the appearance of the batter. Bake at 185°C (365°F) until a toothpick inserted in the center comes out clean (30 to 35 minutes). Place the cakes on a cooling rack and immediately insert a thermometer very carefully to note the final temperature.

PROCEDURE

1. **Method of creaming**

   a. *Cream 30 seconds*—Prepare the basic formula, but cream on the electric mixer for only 30 seconds.

   b. *Cream 2 minutes (control)*—Cream the butter, sugar, and vanilla together for 1 minute. Stop the mixer and scrape the ingredients from the blades and the sides and bottom of the bowl using a rubber spatula. Cream an additional minute before proceeding with the other steps in the basic formula.

c. *Melted butter*—Melt the butter before adding it to the sugar and vanilla. Cream 2 minutes on an electric mixer. Proceed with the remainder of the basic formula procedure.

2. **Addition of flour and milk**

a. *Milk, flour, milk, flour, milk*—Add a third of the milk and stir 50 strokes; add half of the flour mixture and stir 25 strokes. Add a third of the milk and stir 50 strokes before adding the last half of the flour mixture and stirring 25 strokes. Finally, add the remaining third of the milk and stir 75 strokes (total of 225 strokes).

b. *Milk and flour together, 3 additions*—Add a third of the milk and a third of the flour mixture to the creamed mixture. Stir 75 strokes. Add the second third of both the milk and the flour mixture. Stir another 75 strokes. Add the last third of the milk and the flour mixture and stir another 75 strokes (grand total of 225 strokes).

c. *Flour, milk, flour*—Add half the flour mixture to the creamed mixture and stir 75 strokes. Add all of the milk and stir 75 strokes. Add the last half of the flour mixture and stir 75 strokes (total of 225 strokes).

d. *Flour and milk in 1 addition*—To the creamed mixture, add all of the flour mixture and milk. Stir 225 strokes.

3. **Addition of egg**

a. *Egg white foam without sugar*—Use the basic formula, but weigh 16 g yolk and 32 g white. Add the 16 g of egg yolk to the creamed mixture, but do not add the white to the creamed mixture. Continue with the basic formula until the flour mixture and milk have all been added. Then use a rotary eggbeater to quickly beat the 32 g of egg white to the point where the peaks just bend over. With a rubber spatula, transfer the beaten whites to the batter and fold in the foam with as little manipulation as possible. Follow the basic formula directions for baking.

b. *Conventional meringue method*—Use the basic formula, but weigh 16 g of yolk and 32 g of white. Cream half the sugar (75 g) with the fat. Add the 16 g yolk to the creamed mixture. Reserve the 32 g of egg white and the remaining 75 g of sugar until after the flour mixture and milk have been added, as described in the basic formula. With a rotary eggbeater, beat the egg white to the foamy stage. Gradually add remaining sugar to the egg whites while continuing to beat until the peaks just bend over. Transfer the meringue to the batter. With a rubber spatula, fold the meringue into the batter with as little manipulation as possible. Follow the basic formula directions for baking.

c. *Conventional sponge method*—Cream half the sugar (75 g) with the fat. After finishing creaming the sugar, fat, and vanilla, proceed to add the flour mixture and milk, as described in the basic formula. Then beat the whole egg (48 g) until frothy. Gradually add the remaining sugar and continue beating to make the foam as light as possible. Fold this foam into the batter, using a rubber spatula to fold as efficiently as possible. Bake according to the directions in the basic formula.

4. **Muffin method**

a. *Muffin method (control)*—Use the ingredients listed in the basic formula, but do not use the mixing method. To make shortened cakes by the muffin method of mixing, begin by melting the butter. Sift all of the dry ingredients together 3 times to blend them together thoroughly. In a separate bowl, beat the egg and then add the milk and melted butter. Beat just enough to blend. Make a well in the dry ingredients, and pour in all of the liquid ingredients. Beat with an electric mixer on medium speed just until the batter is smooth. If preferred, this can be beaten by hand. Either count the number of strokes used when mixing by hand or time the mixing period on the electric mixer. Do not continue beating after the batter is smooth. Bake according to the directions in the basic formula.

b. *Muffin-meringue method*—Weigh ingredients in the basic formula, but weigh 16 g of yolk, 32 g of white, and weigh the sugar in two measures of 75 g each. Prepare the cake batter according to the directions for the muffin method (procedure 4a), but use only the yolk of the egg (16 g) as a part of the liquid ingredients. Save the egg white for the last step in preparing the batter. The dry ingredient mixture is prepared using only 75 g of sugar, plus the other dry ingredients. The remaining 75 g of sugar is reserved for preparing the egg white meringue. With these adjustments, the muffin method is followed until the batter has been beaten until it is smooth. Then the egg white foam is made, with the sugar being added gradually when the foamy stage is reached, and beating is continued until a peak just bends over. The meringue is folded efficiently and gently into the batter, and the cake is baked according to the basic formula.

5. **Single-stage method**

a. *Single-stage method (control)*—Prepare a cake batter containing the ingredients listed in the basic formula, but use the following method of mixing. All ingredients should be at room temperature before beginning to mix the cake batter. Sift the dry ingredients together three times to mix them thoroughly. Add to the bowl containing all of the other ingredients. Beat for 30 seconds on the low speed of the electric mixer, then for 1.5 minutes (90 seconds) on high speed, and finally another 30 seconds at low speed. Bake the cake as outlined in the basic formula.

b. *Single-stage in two steps*—Prepare the cake batter ingredients (see basic formula), but use the following modifications of the single-stage method. Place the butter, vanilla, and 30 ml milk in the mixing bowl. Sift the dry ingredients together three times before adding them to the mixing bowl. Beat for 1 minute at low speed. Stop the mixer and add the remainder of the milk and eggs. Beat 1.5 minutes (90 seconds) at high speed. Bake as outlined in the basic formula.

c. *Solution method*—This modification of the single-stage method is one of particular merit for commercial baking. The ingredients to be used are stated in the basic formula. Begin the mixing by dissolving the sugar in 60 ml of the milk. Add butter, cake flour, baking powder, and salt. Beat on an electric mixer until the mixture is well aerated. Stop the mixer to add the eggs, vanilla, and remaining 60 ml of milk. Beat just to blend. Bake as described in the basic formula.

6. Pastry-blend method

a. *Pastry-blend method (control)*—Use the ingredients listed in the basic formula. Begin this method by beating the butter and flour together thoroughly. Add the remaining dry ingredients (baking powder, sugar, and salt) and half the milk. Blend thoroughly. Stop the mixer while adding the vanilla, egg, and remaining half of the milk. Beat until smooth. Bake as described in the basic procedure.

EVALUATION

Objective evaluation   Let the cakes cool on wire racks (in an upright position) until cooled to room temperature. Use one of each pair of cakes to determine volume in the volumeter. If time permits, use the penetrometer to assess tenderness.

Subjective evaluation   Although shortened cakes often are iced before being served, there still is interest in evaluating the exterior appearance. Note the general contour of the crust and the browning. To evaluate the interior, look carefully at the cell structure. Look for uniformity of cell size, small cells, and thin cell walls. The texture of shortened cakes is of great importance and is of particular interest when evaluating the cakes made by different mixing methods. To aid in developing the perception of textural characteristics, compare the various cakes carefully. Look for subtle differences, not just gross impressions. Flavor should be evaluated for the total blend of flavor and any indication of aftertaste. Tenderness needs to be evaluated very carefully. Use the number of chews as the measure. Note what correspondence there may be between the subjective and objective evaluations of tenderness.

The keeping quality of cakes needs to be evaluated when considering the merits of different methods. One of the pair of cakes should be stored (tightly covered with plastic wrap) at room temperature for 2 to 5 days and then evaluated subjectively in the same manner as was used for judging the fresh cakes.

If time does not permit evaluation of the fresh cakes on the day they are baked, tightly cover one of the pair of cakes with aluminum foil and freeze for later evaluation. The frozen samples should be thawed completely before being evaluated.

A useful means of recording information about these cakes is to cut a sample of the fresh cake (a slice about 1/2″ thick) and photocopy the cross section. Another technique is to make an inkblot. Unwrap the frozen sample and immediately make an inkblot to record the texture of the cake. The technique is useful in helping to develop the ability to evaluate cake texture.

STUDY QUESTIONS

1. Outline the steps involved in preparing shortened cakes by the conventional method. What is accomplished by each step? Why is it important to control the number of strokes used to mix the batter?

2. Is there any advantage in creaming fat and sugar together longer than the 30 seconds? If so, what is the advantage? What is the purpose of the creaming process? Can it be done effectively when the fat is melted?

3. Contrast the results of the 5 methods used to add the flour and milk in the conventional method. Which method produced the best cake? Did this method require more time than the other methods? If so, was the amount of time required well spent, or is another shorter method almost as satisfactory?

4. Are there advantages to adding eggs as foams? If so, is it beneficial to add sugar to the foam? What effect does sugar have on the meringue and on the cake?

5. Compare the results of mixing by the muffin method with those using the conventional method. How much time does the muffin method save? When would the muffin method be a good method to use?

6. Outline the procedure for the conventional-meringue, conventional-sponge, muffin, muffin-meringue, single-stage, pastry-blend, and solution methods of making shortened cakes. Cite the advantages and disadvantages of each.

7. Describe a shortened cake of high quality.

CHART 10.1.1 DATA ON CAKES MIXED BY DIFFERENT METHODS

Treatment	Strokes (if not 225)	Time to mix	Batter description	Final temperature	Objective testing	
					Volume	Penetrometer
1. Creaming a. 30 sec						
b. 2 min (control)						
c. Melted						
2. Flour, milk addition FMFMF (control) (see 1b) a. MFMFM						
b. MF:3x						
c. FMF						
d. FM:1x						
3. Addition of egg a. White foam, no sugar						
b. White + sugar foam (conv. meringue)						
c. Whole + sugar (conv. sponge)						
4. Muffin a. Control						
b. Meringue						
5. Single-stage a. Control						
b. 2 steps						
c. Solution						
6. Pastry-blend a. Control						

Name

ADDITIONAL OBSERVATIONS AND NOTES

CHART 10.1.2   SUBJECTIVE EVALUATION OF CAKES MIXED BY DIFFERENT METHODS

Treatment	Exterior appearance	Texture			Flavor		Tenderness	
		Uniformity	Cell size	Cell wall	Fresh	Stale	Fresh	Stale
1. Creaming a. 30 sec								
b. 2 min (control)								
c. Melted								
2. Flour, milk addition FMFMF (control) (see 1b) a. MFMFM								
b. MF:3x								
c. FMF								
d. FM:1x								
3. Additional egg a. White foam, no sugar								
b. White + sugar foam (conv. meringue)								
c. Whole + sugar (conv. sponge)								
4. Muffin a. Control								
b. Meringue								
5. Single-stage a. Control								
b. 2 steps								
c. Solution								
6. Pastry-blend a. Control								

Name

ADDITIONAL OBSERVATIONS AND NOTES

EXPERIMENT 10.2—VARYING INGREDIENTS IN SHORTENED CAKES
OBJECTIVES

Upon completion of the experiment, you will be able to:

1. Evaluate cakes and recognize errors that may exist in the formulation of the mixture.
2. Explain the effect of sugar on the volume and tenderness of shortened cakes.
3. Explain the effects on shortened cakes if each of the following is increased: (a) eggs, (b) fat, (c) liquid, and (d) baking powder.
4. Identify the optimum temperature for baking shortened cakes.
5. Interpret the effects of substituting various flours and fats in making shortened cakes.

BASIC FORMULA—SHORTENED CAKE

Full formula	*Half formula*
56 g (1/4 c) Shortening	28 g Shortening
150 g (3/4 c) Sugar	75 g Sugar
3 ml (1/2 tsp) Vanilla	1.5 ml Vanilla
48 g (1) Egg	24 g Egg
150 g (1 1/2 c) Cake flour	75 g Cake flour
5.4 g (1 1/2 tsp) Baking powder	2.7 g Baking powder
2 g (1/4 tsp) Salt	1.0 g Salt
120 ml (1/2 c) Milk	60 ml Milk

Line the bottom of a cake pan (5 3/4″ × 3 1/2″ × 2″) with wax paper cut to fit. Preheat oven to 185°C (365°F).

Cream the shortening, sugar, and vanilla together for 2 minutes on an electric mixer set at the speed indicated for creaming (or on medium if creaming is not indicated). Pour the egg into the mixer and beat 1 minute. Stop the mixer and scrape the beater blades clean with a rubber spatula. Add approximately a third of the mixture of sifted flour, baking powder, and salt. With a wooden spoon, stir the mixture 50 strokes. Add half the milk and stir 25 strokes. Add another third of the flour mixture and stir 50 strokes. Add the last half of the milk and stir 25 strokes. Finally, add the last third of the flour mixture and stir 75 strokes (grand total of 225 strokes). Bake at 185°C (365°F) until a toothpick inserted in the center comes out clean (20 to 25 minutes). Place the cake on a cooling rack and immediately insert a thermometer and record the interior temperature. Note also the baking time. Cool 10 minutes and then remove from the pan for evaluation.

PROCEDURE

1. **Varying the flour**—The various flours on the market have differing characteristics, making some of them more suitable than others for making shortened cakes.

   a. *Cake flour (control)*—Prepare *half* the basic formula.

b. *Cake flour, 90 g*—Prepare *half* the basic formula, but increase the total amount of cake flour to 90 g (20% increase).

c. *All purpose flour*—Prepare *half* the basic formula, but substitute all purpose for cake flour.

d. *Unbleached flour*—Prepare *half* the basic formula, but use unbleached flour in place of cake flour.

e. *Self-rising flour*—Prepare *half* the basic formula, but substitute 77 g self-rising flour for the cake flour and omit the baking powder and salt.

2. **Varying the sugar**—This series is composed of varying levels and types of sugar and sugar products. (**Note:** Full formula [enough for 2 cakes] is made, with each cake being modified according to specific directions.)

a. *225 g sugar (1 1/2 times)*—Prepare the *full* basic formula, but increase sugar to a total of 225 g. Pour 225 g batter into a prepared cake pan. Mix the remaining batter 225 strokes more. Weigh out 225 g batter into the other prepared cake pan and mark it with an X, using a wax marking pencil. Place both pans in the preheated oven and bake according to the basic formula.

b. *300 g sugar (2 times)*—Prepare the *full* basic formula, but increase the sugar to 300 g total. Pour 225 g into a prepared cake pan. Mix the remaining batter 225 more strokes. Weigh out 225 g into the other prepared cake pan and mark it with an X using a wax marking pencil. Place both pans in the preheated oven and bake according to the basic formula directions.

c. *Powdered sugar*—Prepare *half* the basic formula, but substitute powdered sugar for granulated sugar.

d. *Brown sugar*—Prepare *half* the basic formula, but substitute brown sugar for granulated sugar.

e. *Sucralose*—Prepare *half* the basic formula, but omit the sugar and add 9 g sucralose.

f. *Honey*—Prepare *half* the basic formula, but reduce the milk to 30 ml, omit the sugar, and substitute with 90 ml honey.

3. **Varying eggs**—In this series the amount of egg and the type of egg are varied to show their effects.

a. *48 g egg (2 times)*—Prepare *half* the basic formula, but add a total of 48 g egg.

b. *Egg substitute*—Prepare *half* the basic formula, but use 24 g egg substitute in place of the egg.

4. **Fat modifications**—In this series, the levels of fat are modified, mixing time is tested in conjunction with the changes in fat levels, and the types of fats also are tested. Note that *full* formula (2 cakes) is prepared for variations a and b, with each cake being modified according to directions.

a. *84 g shortening (1.5 times)*—Prepare the *full* basic formula, but increase the shortening to 84 g total. Weigh out 225 g batter into prepared pan. Mix the remaining batter 225 strokes. Weigh out 225 g batter into prepared pan marked with an X. Place both pans in the oven and bake.

b. *112 g shortening (2 times)*—Prepare the *full* basic formula, but increase the total amount of shortening to 112 g. Weigh out 225 g batter into a prepared pan. Mix the remaining batter 225 strokes. Weigh out 225 g batter into the prepared pan marked with an X. Place both pans in the oven and bake.

c. *Oil*—Prepare *half* the basic formula, but substitute salad oil for shortening. Beat the oil with the sugar to incorporate as much air as possible.

d. *Margarine*—Prepare *half* the basic formula, but substitute margarine for shortening.

e. *Butter*—Prepare *half* the basic formula, but substitute butter for shortening.

f. *Flax seed*—Prepare *half* the basic formula, but reduce shortening to 14 g and add 24 g ground flax seed.

5. **Baking temperatures**—Baking temperatures significantly higher or lower than recommended are used in this series to demonstrate the importance of temperature control on shortened cakes. This series is to be prepared by one group; the results are to be compared with the control cake 1a when evaluation is being done. Directions for preparing this series are as follows: Prepare the *full* basic formula. Weigh out 225 g batter into a prepared cake pan (for variation a), and weigh 225 g batter into another prepared cake pan (for variation b).

a. *150°C (300°F)*—Bake 1 cake in an oven preheated to 150°C.

b. *204°C (400°F)*—Bake 1 cake in an oven preheated to 204°C.

6. **Other variables**

a. *75 ml milk (25% increase)*—Prepare *half* the basic formula, but increase the milk to 75 ml.

b. *5.4 g baking powder (2 times)*—Prepare *half* the basic formula, but increase the baking powder to a total of 5.4 g.

EVALUATION

Objective evaluation   Determine the volume by using the volumeter on each cake. Since the cakes will also be used for subjective testing, wrap tightly in a single layer of plastic wrap before testing. Test the tenderness objectively with the penetrometer. Then the cake is ready for use in subjective testing.

Subjective evaluation   Sensory evaluation is done after the objective tests are completed. The variations tested in different parts of the experiment will have some distinctly different effects on exterior appearance, texture, color, flavor, and tenderness of the cakes. Careful attention to evaluating these aspects is very important.

STUDY QUESTIONS

1. Describe each of the cakes made with the following flours: all purpose, unbleached, and self-rising. Compare them with the control cake that was made with cake flour. Would any of these flours make a satisfactory substitute for cake flour?

2. What effect does increasing the level of sugar have on the volume of a shortened cake? What is the effect on the temperature of coagulation? Does mixing need to be modified when the level of sugar is increased? If so, how?

3. What effect(s) can be observed when the level of egg in a cake is increased? Is the change (as demonstrated in this experiment) desirable? Explain your answer.

4. When making a shortened cake, can powdered sugar be substituted satisfactorily for granulated sugar on a weight basis? Can (a) brown sugar or (b) a sugar substitute be substituted for granulated sugar when making a shortened cake? Explain your answers for each of these substitutions.

5. What changes are needed when honey is substituted for sugar in a shortened cake? Why are these changes necessary?

6. Can an egg substitute be used in a shortened cake to replace an egg? Why?

7. What is the effect of increasing the amount of fat in a shortened cake? What effect does this increase have on the amount of mixing recommended for optimum structure?

8. Which fats and oil were satisfactory replacements for shortening? Describe the effects of each fat and oil used.

9. Can flax seeds be substituted satisfactorily for part of the fat in a shortened cake? Describe the cake produced in this variation.

10. What effect(s) did increasing the level of milk have on a shortened cake?

11. How critical is the baking temperature for shortened cake? What effects, if any, were observed as a result of using (a) too low and (b) too high an oven temperature?

CHART 10.2.1   EVALUATION OF SHORTENED CAKES MADE WITH VARYING INGREDIENTS

Treatment	Baking time	Interior temp.	Volume (ml)	Penetrometer (mm)
1. Flour				
a. Cake flour (Control)				
b. 20% increase				
c. All purpose				
d. Unbleached				
e. Self-rising				
2. Sugar				
a. 1 1/2x, 225x				
1 1/2x, 450x				
b. 2x, 225x				
2x, 450x				
c. Powdered				
d. Brown				
e. Sucralose				
f. Honey				
3. Eggs				
a. 2x				
b. Substitute				
4. Fat				
a. 1 1/2x, 225x				
1 1/2x, 450x				
b. 2x, 225x				
2x, 450x				
c. Oil				
d. Margarine				
e. Butter				
f. Flax seed				
5. Temperature				
a. 150°C				
b. 204°C				
6. Other				
a. +25% milk				
b. 2x baking powder				

Name

ADDITIONAL OBSERVATIONS AND NOTES

CHART 10.2.2 SUBJECTIVE EVALUATION OF SHORTENED CAKES WITH VARYING INGREDIENTS

Treatment	Exterior appearance	Texture Cell size	Cell wall	Color (# chews)	Flavor	Tenderness
1. Flour						
a. Cake flour (control)						
b. 20% increase						
c. All purpose						
d. Unbleached						
e. Self-rising						
2. Sugar						
a. 1 1/2x, 225x						
1 1/2x, 450x						
b. 2x, 225x						
2x, 450x						
c. Powdered						
d. Brown						
e. Sucralose						
f. Honey						
3. Eggs						
a. 2x						
b. Substitute						
4. Fat						
a. 1 1/2x, 225x						
1 1/2x, 450x						
b. 2x, 225x						
2x, 450x						
c. Oil						
d. Margarine						
e. Butter						
f. Flax seed						
5. Temperature						
a. 150°C						
b. 204°C						
6. Other						
a. +25% milk						
b. 2x baking powder						

Name

ADDITIONAL OBSERVATIONS AND NOTES

11
Pastry

Pie is a favorite type of American dessert. Although only four ingredients are used in the pastry, the quality of the crusts made with these ingredients varies widely from one cook to another. The quality of the pastry is critical to producing a satisfactory pie and should be evaluated independently, with the filling being considered separately. Quality of pastry is judged primarily on two characteristics: flakiness and tenderness.

When the overall quality of a pie is being judged, soaking of the crust is one factor that needs to be considered. This may be a particular problem in one-crust pies with custard-type fillings. The upper crust of a two-crust pie offers additional potential risk for sogginess because of trapped steam generated during baking.

The experiments in this chapter are directed toward determining factors influencing the quality of pastry. Ways of reducing problems with sogginess are explored, too. The knowledge gained in this chapter can be combined usefully with the information gained from the experiment on fats in pastry in Chapter 4.

EXPERIMENT 11.1—FACTORS INFLUENCING PASTRY QUALITY
OBJECTIVES

Upon completion of the experiment, you will be able to:

1. Evaluate the quality of pastry.
2. Identify variables in making pastry that promote tenderness and those that promote toughness.
3. Identify variables in pastry making that promote flakiness.
4. Evaluate the merits of using different methods of making pastry and of using different liquids.

BASIC FORMULA—PASTRY

87 g (3/4 c)	All purpose flour
47 g (1/4 c)	Shortening
29.5 ml (2 tbsp)	Water
1.5 g (1/4 tsp)	Salt

Add salt to flour and stir briefly with a 4-tined fork. Add fat all at once. Use a pastry blender to cut the fat into pieces the size of uncooked rice grains. Sprinkle the water over the surface of the mixture, a drop at a time, while flipping the mixture lightly with a 4-tined fork. Continue sprinkling and flipping actions until all of the water has been added.

With the fork, mash the dough together to make a ball (use approximately 10 strokes). Avoid extra manipulation. Turn the ball out onto a piece of wax paper about 12″ long. Very quickly manipulate the dough in the wax paper into a cohesive ball. Avoid holding this in the hands any longer than necessary to form the ball so the dough will not be warmed unduly. Arrange a strip of wax paper on a special bread board equipped with parallel guides so that the wax paper just covers the area between the guides. Quickly shape the dough into a flattened oblong shape on the wax paper strip, and place another wax paper strip on top. Lightly roll the dough until it is the thickness of the guides. Remove any dough that spreads onto the guides and add it to the ends of the dough being rolled. Keep rolling until no more dough spreads onto the guides and the dough is a uniform thickness. Remove the top piece of wax paper, and use a rectangular cutter to efficiently cut as many rectangles as possible. Invert a baking sheet over the pastry board and flip the sheet and board quickly to transfer the rectangles of pastry to the baking sheet. Remove the wax paper and the dough between the rectangles. Prick the surface of the rectangles with a fork to minimize blistering during baking. Bake at 218°(425°F) until a pleasing, light golden brown. Note the baking time required.

PROCEDURE

1. **Variations in the amount of water**—Although the crusts will vary in their ease of handling, attempt to handle and manipulate them precisely, according to the basic formula.

   a. *25 ml water*—Prepare the basic formula, but reduce the water to 25 ml total.

   b. *29.5 ml water (control)*—Prepare the basic formula. This will serve as the control for the entire experiment.

   c. *35 ml water*—Prepare the basic formula, but increase the water to a total of 35 ml.

2. **Amount of mixing**

   a. *No stirring*—Prepare the basic formula, but do not stir the dough after the water has been added. Instead, immediately transfer all of the dough to wax paper and work it with the hands just enough to make the dough stay together for rolling.

   b. *Stir 25 times*—Prepare the basic formula, but stir the dough 25 times total before proceeding to the next step in preparing the dough.

3. **Chilling dough**

  a. *10 minutes in freezer*—After dough has been stirred and worked into a ball, wrap the ball in aluminum foil. Store in the freezer for 10 minutes. Note the temperature at the center of the dough when it is removed from the freezer. Proceed with the rolling according to the basic formula.

  b. *30 minutes in refrigerator*—Prepare basic formula as in procedure 3a, but chill the dough 30 minutes in the refrigerator. Note the temperature in the center of the dough when the ball is removed.

4. **Temperature of liquid**

  a. *Ice water*—Prepare a bowl of ice water and let it cool until the temperature remains constant. Prepare the basic formula, but use the ice water as the liquid.

  b. *Chipped ice*—Place an ample amount of ice in a blender and whirl it until the ice is in fine pieces. Weigh 29.5 g chipped ice. Prepare the basic formula, using the weighed chipped ice as the liquid. Add into the dough any of the water that may collect from the melting ice after the ice has been weighed.

  c. *Boiling water*—Prepare the basic formula, but beat the water (use boiling water) and fat together by hand before stirring in the dry ingredients. Follow the directions in the basic formula for shaping, rolling, and baking.

  d. *Boiling water, chilled dough*—Prepare dough as described in procedure 4c, but wrap the dough in aluminum foil and chill 10 minutes in the refrigerator. Measure the temperature of the center of the dough when the ball is removed from the refrigerator. Follow the directions for the basic formula for shaping, rolling, and baking.

5. **Liquids**

  a. *Orange juice*—Prepare the basic formula, but substitute orange juice for water.

  b. *Milk*—Prepare the basic formula, but substitute milk for the water.

  c. *Cream*—Prepare the basic formula, but substitute cream for water.

6. **Handling during rolling**—When dough does not roll into the desired shape, the temptation is strong to re-roll the crust into the right shape. This not a problem for those experienced in making pastry, but is of interest to those who lack experience in this product. This series demonstrates the results of re-rolling dough.

  a. *Re-roll dough 1 time*—Prepare the basic formula, but after rolling dough to the correct thickness, pick up the dough and work it into a ball. Roll it out again before proceeding with the cutting and baking.

  b. *Re-roll 2 times*—Prepare the basic formula, as described in 6a, but shape the dough into a ball and re-roll a second time before proceeding with the cutting and baking.

c. *Re-roll 3 times*—Prepare the basic formula, as described in procedure 6b, but shape and re-roll the dough a third time before proceeding with the cutting and baking.

EVALUATION

Objective evaluation   Evaluate tenderness objectively using the shortometer. Measure the height (in mm) of a stack of 3 pastry wafers to evaluate flakiness objectively.

Subjective evaluation   Subjectively evaluate color, flavor, tenderness, and flakiness.

STUDY QUESTIONS

1. Describe a pastry of high quality. What factors determine whether or not a pastry will meet this standard?

2. What change(s) can be observed as the amount of water in a pastry is increased? What may influence how much water may be needed in a pastry to achieve optimum quality?

3. What changes take place as mixing is increased? What happens as re-rolling is increased?

4. Does chilling the dough influence the final quality of a pastry? If so, how?

5. Does the use of different liquids modify the characteristics of the crust? If so, how?

6. Are there benefits from using liquid at a particular temperature (or approximate temperature)? Describe the pastry made with boiling water.

CHART 11.1   EVALUATION OF PASTRY MADE WITH VARYING METHODS AND INGREDIENTS

Treatment	Short-ometer	Ht. of 3 layers (mm)	Color	Flavor	Tenderness	Flakiness
1. Amount of water a. 25 ml						
b. 29.5 ml (control)						
c. 35 ml						
2. Mixing a. No stir						
b. 25 x						
3. Chilling a. 10 min. in freezer (temp. ___°C)						
b. 30 min. in refrig. (temp. ___°C)						
4. Temp. of liquid a. Ice water						
b. Chipped ice						
c. Boiling water						
d. Boiling water, chilled (temp. ___°C)						
5. Liquids a. Orange juice						
b. Milk						
c. Cream						
6. Re-rolling a. 1x						
b. 2x						
c. 3x						

Name

ADDITIONAL OBSERVATIONS AND NOTES

EXPERIMENT 11.2—FACTORS INFLUENCING SOAKING OF PASTRY OBJECTIVES

Upon completion of the experiment, you will be able to:

1. Evaluate two-crust pies, with particular emphasis on evaluation of the crusts.
2. Identify techniques that are helpful in minimizing the soaking of pie crusts.

BASIC FORMULA—CRUST

2-crust pie	*1-crust pie*
110 g (1c) All purpose flour	55 g All purpose flour
3 g (1/4 tsp) Salt	1.5 g Salt
66 g (1/3 c) Shortening	33 g Shortening
40 ml (1/6 c) Water	20 ml Water

Stir flour and salt together with a 4-tined fork. Add shortening and cut in with a pastry blender until pieces are the size of uncooked rice grains. Toss the flour mixture lightly with a fork while slowly adding the water. After all of the water is added, stir approximately 10 strokes with the fork until the dough forms into a ball. If making 2 crusts, divide the dough into 2 balls of approximately equal size. Roll one of the balls into a circle of dough 1/8" thick, using the special guides to control thickness.

Fold the rolled dough in quarters. Unfold in a 5" pie plate, adjusting to fit up the sides without stretching the dough. For a 1-crust pie, trim 1/2" beyond the edge of the pie plate and flute the dough so that it rests on the lip of the plate.

For a 2-crust pie, trim the dough of the bottom crust even with the edge of the pie plate. Roll the second crust in the same manner as the first. Fold this upper crust in quarters and set aside until the filling (see basic formula—cherry pie) has been prepared and placed in the bottom crust. Unfold the second crust and adjust over the filling so that the edges extend beyond the lip of the pie plate. Trim the top crust 1/2" beyond the edge of the pie plate. Fold this extension under the bottom crust that is resting on the lip of the plate; flute the dough "sandwich" so it rests on the lip of the pie plate. With a paring knife, cut a design of slits each about 1/2" long in the center region of the upper crust. Bake in a preheated oven at 218°C (425°F) for approximately 20 minutes, until the crust is golden and the juice begins to bubble (as seen through the slits in the top crust).

BASIC FORMULA—CHERRY PIE FILLING

35 g	Sugar
2 g	Cornstarch
60 ml	Juice drained from canned cherries
130 g	Canned sour pie cherries, pitted and drained
5 g	Butter or margarine

Stir the sugar and cornstarch together in a heavy saucepan. Slowly stir in the juice with a wooden spoon. Heat over direct heat, stirring constantly, until the mixture comes to a rolling boil. Remove from the heat, and stir in the cherries and butter. Pour into the bottom crust.

PROCEDURE

1. **Treatments of the bottom crust**—Various techniques can be considered as possible solutions to the problem of a soaked crust.

   a. *Hot filling (control)*—Prepare pastry for a 2-crust pie and cherry pie filling. Pour hot filling into bottom crust. Bake as in the basic formula.

   b. *Coat bottom crust with butter*—Prepare pastry for 2-crust pie and cherry pie filling. Brush soft butter all across the bottom crust to serve as a seal before adding the pie filling. Bake as in the basic formula.

   c. *Brush with egg white*—Prepare pastry for 2-crust pie and cherry pie filling. Brush slightly beaten egg white foam on the surface of the bottom crust before adding the filling. Also, brush slightly-beaten egg white foam on the bottom side of the upper crust before it is placed on top of the filling. Bake as in the basic formula.

   d. *Cold filling*—Prepare pastry for 2-crust pie and cherry pie filling as described above, but chill the filling in the refrigerator to 25°C before placing it in the unbaked bottom crust and proceeding with the basic formula.

2. **Thickness of crust**

   a. *Crust 1/4" thick*—Prepare pastry for 2-crust pie and cherry filling, but roll the crusts 1/4" thick. Bake according to the basic formula.

   b. *Crust 1/4" thick, no slits in top crust*—Prepare pastry for 2-crust pie and cherry pie filling, but be sure to roll crust 1/4" thick. Do not cut slits in the top crust. Bake according to the basic formula.

   c. *Crust 3/8" thick*—Prepare pastry for 2-crust pie and cherry pie filling, but use a special board to roll crusts 3/8" thick. Bake according to the basic formula.

3. **Baking conditions**

   a. *150°C (300°F)*—Prepare pastry for 2-crust pie and cherry pie filling, but bake in a preheated oven at 150°C (300°F).

b. *175°C (350°F)*—Prepare pastry for 2-crust pie and cherry pie filling, but bake in a preheated oven at 175°C (350°F).

c. *232°C (450°F)*—Prepare pastry for 2-crust pie and cherry filling, but bake in a preheated oven at 232°C (450°F).

BASIC FORMULA—CUSTARD PIE FILLING

72 g (1 1/2)	Egg
236 ml (1 c)	Milk
25 g (2 tbsp)	Sugar
2 ml (1/3 tsp)	Vanilla

Beat egg gently with a rotary eggbeater until uniformly blended. Scald milk to 65°C. Add milk, sugar, and vanilla to egg and stir until blended. Pour into an unbaked pie shell and bake at 175°C (350°F) until mixture is set to the point where a knife inserted halfway between the center and the edge of the pie comes out clean.

---

4. Variations in filling treatment

a. *Baked crust, baked filling*—Prepare 1 crust using the basic formula. Be sure to puncture the crust well with a 4-tined fork before baking. Bake the pastry at 218°C (425°F) for about 12 minutes until golden brown. Prepare the basic custard filling, but bake the filling in a buttered pie plate without a crust. Carefully place the pan containing the custard filling in a larger pan containing 1/3" of very hot water. Place this assembly in a preheated oven at 163°C (325°F) and bake until a knife inserted halfway between the center and the edge comes out clean. Let the custard cool in its pan after carefully removing it from the water bath. When the custard pan is slightly warmer than body temperature, carefully slide the custard into the unfilled baked pastry.

b. *Hot filling*—Prepare 1 crust using the basic pastry formula, but do not bake it and do not puncture it with a fork. Prepare filling using the basic formula for a custard pie filling. Pour into unbaked pie shell. Bake as in basic formula for custard pie filling.

c. *Cold filling*—Prepare 1 crust using the basic pastry formula, but do not bake and do not puncture with a fork. Prepare filling using the basic formula for a custard pie filling, but let it cool to room temperature and then pour into the unbaked pastry shell. Bake as in basic formula for custard pie filling.

d. *Partially baked crust*—Prepare filling as in basic custard formula. Prepare the crust as described in the 1-crust pastry formula, but do not assemble the pie until the pastry has been punctured with a 4-tined fork to avoid blistering and then baked 4 minutes in a preheated oven at 218°C (425°F). Then the filling is poured in, and the pie is baked according to the basic formula for custard pie.

e. *Baked crust, hot filling*—Prepare the basic 1-crust pastry formula, but bake the punctured crust for 12 minutes until golden brown in a preheated oven at 218°C (425°F). Prepare the custard filling and pour the hot filling into the baked crust. Bake the pie according to the directions in the custard pie filling basic formula.

5. **Baking temperatures**

a. *150°C (300°F)*—Prepare 1-crust basic pastry and custard pie filling, but bake in a preheated oven at 150°C.

b. *204°C (400°F)*—Prepare 1-crust pastry and custard pie filling, but bake in a preheated oven at 204°C.

c. *Microwave oven*—Prepare 1-crust pastry formula. Place in a glass baking dish, puncture crust, and bake for 2 minutes in a microwave oven. Add custard pie filling and heat in a microwave oven another 3 minutes. Let stand briefly to cool before evaluating.

EVALUATION

Subjective evaluation   Subjective evaluation is the preferred means of testing the results of these variations. The point of greatest concern is the bottom crust in most of the samples. For the cherry pie sample in which the upper crust was not slit (procedure 2b), note the condition of the upper crust and compare it with the cherry pies that had slits in the upper crust. The point of evaluation is the crispness or the sogginess of the crusts. Consider also the palatability of the fillings.

STUDY QUESTIONS

1. Are there any ways of preventing a soggy crust in pies? Does it help to cut slits in the top crust of a two-crust pie?

2. What way(s) of preparing the bottom crust of a pie seemed to be effective in minimizing soaking of the bottom crust?

3. Is there a relationship between the tendency of a crust to soak up liquid from the filling and the thickness of the crust? Explain your answer.

4. Does baking temperature influence the soaking of a crust?

5. Based on the results of this experiment, is it possible to prepare custard pies satisfactorily using the microwave oven?

CHART 11.2.1   EVALUATION OF SOAKING OF PIE CRUSTS —CHERRY PIE

Treatment	Condition of crust		Filling palatability
	Bottom	**Top**	
1. Treat bottom crust a. Hot filling (control)			
b. Coat with butter			
c. Coat, egg white			
d. Cold filling			
2. Thickness of crust a. 1/4″			
b. 1/4″, no slit in top			
c. 3/8″			
3. Baking conditions a. 150°C (300°F)			
b. 175°C (350°F)			
c. 232°C (450°F)			

Name

ADDITIONAL OBSERVATIONS AND NOTES

CHART 11.2.2 EVALUATION OF SOAKING OF PIE CRUSTS—CUSTARD PIE

Treatment	Condition of crust	Filling palatability
4. Variation, filling a. Baked crust, baked filling		
b. Hot filling, unbaked crust		
c. Cold filling, unbaked crust		
d. Partially baked crust		
e. Baked crust		
5. Temperatures a. 150°C (300°F)		
b. 204°C (400°F)		
c. Microwave oven		

Name

ADDITIONAL OBSERVATIONS AND NOTES

12

Food Preservation

Although many people today rely on the food industry to preserve foods for later use, food also may be preserved at home. Preservation may be by reducing the moisture content significantly, as is done in drying and freeze-drying. Another means of prolonging shelf life of foods is by adding relatively high concentrations of sugar or salt, both of which are effective in inhibiting the growth of microorganisms that can make food unsafe to eat. Temperature, either high enough or very cold, can be altered during processing and/or storage to preserve foods.

Freezing and canning are common ways of preserving foods today. Freezing is effective because low storage temperatures, preferably at $-18°C$ (0°F) or below, significantly inhibit the growth of microorganisms. Canning is an effective means of preserving because the high temperature reached during the heat processing kills microorganisms that might have been present prior to canning. All of these methods are safe when done properly, and they can be done in the home. However, careful attention must be given to such key factors as temperature control and sugar concentrations if preserved foods are to be safe when they are eaten after storage.

Experiments on canning are omitted from this manual to avoid health risks that could result from experiments involving variations in canning techniques and conditions. The experiments on freezing, drying, and jelly making serve to illustrate some of the principles involved in preserving foods safely.

EXPERIMENT 12.1—PRESERVING BY FREEZING
OBJECTIVES

Upon completion of the experiment, you will be able to:

1. Explain the reasons for blanching vegetables prior to freezing.
2. Evaluate the various types of containers available for freezing foods.
3. Discuss the changes that take place in the structure of various foods during the freezing process and in frozen storage.
4. Identify means of enhancing the quality of frozen food products.
5. Discuss the role of food additives (sugar, salt, and ascorbic acid, for example) in the freezing of foods.

BASIC FORMULA—FROZEN BROCCOLI

1/3 lb Broccoli

Trim stalks and wash thoroughly. Soak for 30 minutes in salt water (1 qt water and 1 tsp salt). Remove from water and split stalks lengthwise. In a kettle large enough to accommodate the blanching basket, bring enough water to a boil to cover the broccoli in the basket. When the water is boiling actively, place the broccoli in the basket and immerse the vegetable. Maintain an active boil throughout the entire 3-minute blanching period. Immediately immerse the broccoli in ice water for 3 minutes. Drain thoroughly and pack broccoli carefully and efficiently into a plastic freezer container (labeled with the variation and the date). Immediately place the container in the freezer.

PROCEDURE

1. **Freezing vegetables**

   a. *Blanching time 1 minute*—Prepare the basic formula, but blanch only 1 minute and chill in ice water only 1 minute.

   b. *Blanching time 3 minutes (control)*—Prepare the basic formula.

   c. *Blanching time 5 minutes*—Prepare basic formula, but blanch 5 minutes and chill in ice water for 5 minutes.

   d. *Unblanched*—Prepare as in basic formula, but do not blanch the vegetable and do not chill in ice water.

   e. *Water pack*—Prepare as in basic formula, but pour enough of the blanching water (cooled) over the broccoli to cover the vegetable in the container.

   f. *Salt added*—Prepare the basic formula, but blanch in salt water (1 tsp salt/qt water).

   g. *Glass jar*—Prepare the basic formula, but pack in a glass freezer jar.

h. *Uncovered*—Prepare the basic formula, but freeze in an uncovered container.

i. *Aluminum foil*—Prepare the basic formula, but wrap broccoli in heavy aluminum foil, being careful to fold all seams at least twice to seal tightly.

j. *Plastic bag*—Prepare the basic formula, but place the broccoli in a plastic bag. Press air from the bag before zipping or twisting several times to minimize the air in the package during storage.

k. *Room temperature cooling*—Prepare the basic formula, but allow the blanched broccoli to cool slowly to room temperature before freezing.

l. *No cooling*—Prepare the basic formula, but package and freeze immediately after blanching.

m. *Ice pack*—Prepare the basic formula, but place the plastic freezer container in an ice pack for 1 hour before transferring it to the freezer.

n. *1 c salt, 1 qt ice*—Prepare the basic formula, but place the plastic freezer container in an ice pack made by stirring together 1 c rock salt and 1 qt crushed ice. Chill 1 hour before placing in the freezer. Measure the temperature of the ice water formed at the end of 30 minutes and 60 minutes.

2. **Freezing fruits**

a. *No sugar or syrup*—Wash, sort, and hull 1/2 pt strawberries. Drain well before placing in a freezer container. Cover tightly and freeze at once.

b. *Dry sugar pack*—Repeat 2a, but sprinkle 40 g sugar over the strawberries after they are drained and placed in a plastic freezer container. Very gently stir them to dissolve the sugar. Cover tightly and freeze at once.

c. *30% sugar syrup*—Prepare syrup by boiling 1 c sugar with 2 c water just until the sugar dissolves. Cool the syrup while preparing the berries as in 2a. Pour 125 ml of the cooled sugar syrup (30% concentration) into the freezer container. Add the berries and shake very gently to settle them efficiently into the container. Add additional liquid syrup to cover the berries, being sure to leave at least 1/2″ head space. Cover tightly and freeze at once.

d. *50% sugar syrup*—Prepare syrup by boiling 2 c sugar with 2 c water just until the sugar dissolves and then cooling it. Prepare berries as in 2a. Pour 125 ml of the cooled syrup into a freezer container. Add the berries and shake gently to settle the berries efficiently. Add syrup to cover the berries, being sure to leave at least 1/2″ head space. Cover tightly and freeze immediately.

e. *Sucralose*—Prepare as in 2a, but sprinkle 4.8 g sucralose on the berries in a plastic freezer container, and stir carefully to dissolve it over all of the berries. Cover tightly and freeze immediately.

f. *Apples or pears, no ascorbic acid, dry sugar*—Wash, pare, and slice 1 apple (or pear). Place in freezer container and sprinkle 15 g sugar over the slices. Stir gently to coat the fruit. Cover tightly and freeze immediately.

g. *Apples or pears, ascorbic acid, dry sugar*—Wash, pare, and slice 1 apple (or pear). Place in a freezer container. Dissolve 1/8 tsp ascorbic acid in 5 ml water and pour over the fruit. Sprinkle 15 g sugar over the slices and stir gently to coat the fruit. Cover tightly and freeze immediately.

h. *Cantaloupe*—Cut melon in half, remove the seeds, and carve into melon balls. Place the balls in a plastic freezer container. Cover tightly and freeze immediately.

3. **Freezing eggs**

a. *Whole eggs, no additives*—Gently beat 1 egg to blend until homogeneous, but not foamy. Pour into a small plastic container or bag. Cover tightly and freeze immediately.

b. *Whole egg, 0.5 g salt*—Prepare as in 3a, but add 0.5 g salt before beating.

c. *Whole egg, 4 g sugar*—Prepare as in 3a, but add 4 g sugar before beating.

d. *Yolk, no additives*—Beat 1 egg yolk slightly and freeze in a plastic bag or container.

e. *Yolk, 0.2 g salt*—Add 0.2 g salt to 1 egg yolk and beat slightly. Freeze in a plastic bag or container.

f. *Yolk, 1.5 g sugar*—Add 1.5 g sugar to 1 egg yolk and beat slightly. Freeze in a plastic bag or container.

g. *White, no additives*—Place 1 egg white in a plastic container or bag and freeze.

h. *White, 0.3 g salt*— Add 0.3 g salt to 1 egg white. Beat just enough to dissolve the salt. Freeze in a plastic bag or container.

i. *White, 2.5 g sugar*—Add 2.5 g sugar to 1 egg white. Beat just enough to dissolve the sugar. Freeze in a plastic bag or container.

EVALUATION

1. If possible, maintain the broccoli in frozen storage for at least a month before evaluating it. When ready to evaluate, cook each treatment of broccoli in a separate 1-qt saucepan by bringing 1/2 c water and 1 g salt to a boil before adding the broccoli and boiling 2 minutes. Drain and serve for evaluation. To evaluate broccoli, note the color and distinctness of its outline. Note the mouthfeel and flavor of the cooked vegetable. A primary characteristic to be evaluated is the integrity of the cell walls. This can be determined by a combination of visual assessment and mouthfeel.

2. After at least a month of storage, remove the fruits from the freezer. Judge their appearance after 30 minutes of thawing uncovered at

room temperature. Remove half of each variation for taste evaluation while the fruit still has ice crystals in it. Evaluate the second half after the fruit has thawed completely. Note particularly the integrity of the cells, any textural changes, and the amount of drip loss exuding from the thawing fruit.

3. If necessary, eggs can be evaluated after as little as a week of frozen storage. Thaw each package completely before evaluating. Examine each treatment by placing in a separate dish and then allowing a spoonful of the egg to flow from the spoon back into the dish. After all students have observed these flow characteristics, each sample of whole egg is scrambled without adding any salt. The flavor and texture of the scrambled egg variations are evaluated subjectively. Each of the yolk samples is used to make a mayonnaise. The yolks are evaluated on the ease of forming the emulsion and its stability. The whites are each evaluated by beating to a foam with peaks that just bend over. Each of the foams is placed in a funnel positioned over a graduated cylinder. The drainage is measured after 15 minutes.

STUDY QUESTIONS

1. What are the differences in the method used for freezing vegetables and that used for freezing fruit? Why are the methods used?

2. What differences can be observed in broccoli prepared for freezing with differing blanching times? What is the result of freezing a vegetable without blanching?

3. Is it essential to cool the vegetable quickly following blanching? Why?

4. Is it wise to add salt to the blanching water? Should vegetables be salted before freezing? Explain your answers.

5. Discuss the advantages and disadvantages of plastic freezer containers, glass freezing containers, aluminum foil, and plastic bags as freezing containers.

6. What method of freezing broccoli in the experiment resulted in maintenance of the best texture in the thawed, cooked product? Explain your choice.

7. Compare the thawed characteristics of strawberries frozen without sugar, with dry sugar pack, with 30% sugar syrup, and with 50% sugar syrup.

8. What is the reason for using ascorbic acid when freezing apples (or pears)? Is it necessary to use it in freezing strawberries? Explain your answer.

9. Describe the characteristics of (a) frozen cantaloupe and (b) strawberries while ice crystals are still present. Describe their characteristics after they are thawed completely.

10. Which treatments for freezing (a) whole egg, (b) yolk, and (c) white gave acceptable results? Explain how each acceptable frozen product could be used satisfactorily in preparing specific dishes. Discuss any factors that influence the use of these frozen egg products.

CHART 12.1.1   FROZEN VEGETABLES—BROCCOLI

Treatment	Appearance	Color	Mouthfeel	Flavor
Blanching time a. 1 min				
b. 3 min (control)				
c. 5 min				
d. Unblanched				
e. Water pack				
f. Salt in blanch water				
Containers g. Glass				
h. Uncovered				
i. Aluminum foil				
j. Plastic bag				
Prepack, cooling k. Room				
l. No cooling				
Freezing temperature m. Ice pack				
n. 1 c salt, 1 qt ice _____°C, 30 min _____°C, 1 hr				

Name _____

ADDITIONAL OBSERVATIONS AND NOTES

CHART 12.1.2   FROZEN FRUITS

Treatment	Appearance		Color	Texture and mouthfeel		Drip loss
	30 min	Thawed		Ice crystals	Thawed	
Strawberries a. No sugar						
b. Dry sugar pack						
c. 30% sugar syrup						
d. 50% sugar syrup						
e. Sugar substitute						
Apples (or pears) f. No ascorbic acid						
g. Ascorbic acid						
h. **Cantaloupe**						

ADDITIONAL OBSERVATIONS AND NOTES

CHART 12.1.3   FROZEN EGGS

Treatment	Flow quality, thawed	Evaluation product	
		Ease of use	**Performance**
Whole egg a. No additive		(in scrambled eggs)	(Flavor, texture)
b. 0.5 g salt			
c. 4 g sugar			
Yolk d. No additive		(in mayonnaise)	(Stability, texture)
e. 0.2 g salt			
f. 1.5 g sugar			
White g. No additive		(in Foam, beating time)	(Drainage, texture)
h. 0.3 g salt			
i. 2.5 g sugar			

Name

ADDITIONAL OBSERVATIONS AND NOTES

EXPERIMENT 12.2—DRYING OF FOODS
OBJECTIVES

Upon completion of the experiment, you will be able to:

1. Identify the reasons for the procedures used in drying fruits and vegetables.
2. Explain the reason for blanching some vegetables and the reason for not blanching other vegetables and fruits.
3. Compare the cost and the quality of home-dried with commercially dried fruits.
4. Evaluate the use of ascorbic acid in retaining color in dried products.
5. Compare the quality of products dried under the conditions tested in the experiment.

PROCEDURE

1. **Drying of onions**—Wash onions, cut off both ends and remove the outer layers of skin. Cut in slices 1/4" thick and separate the layers in each slice. Use 1/2 onion for each of the following treatments.

   a. *Blanch, dry at 140°F (60°C)*—Place onion slices in a basket and boil 2 minutes. Remove and drain on paper towels. Spread slices on cheesecloth stretched tightly across a jelly roll pan, and heat in oven at 140°F until brittle. Note the time required (estimate is 6 hours). Store in a tightly closed container.

   b. *Unblanched, dry at 140° F (60°C)*—Distribute onion slices on cheesecloth spread tightly across a jelly roll pan; dry in 140°F oven until brittle. Note time. Store in a tightly closed container.

   c. *Unblanched, dry at 250°F (121°C)*—Prepare as in 1b, but dry in an oven at 250°F. Note total time required to the point of being brittle. Store in a tightly covered container.

   d. *Unblanched, dehydrator*—Prepare as in 1b, but dry in dehydrator at 140°F.

2. **Drying parsley**—Wash parsley thoroughly and drain on paper towels. Divide bunch into thirds for use in the three treatments that follow. Remove all the long stems before proceeding with each treatment.

   a. *Unblanched, dry at 140°F (60°C)*—Spread parsley on cheesecloth stretched tightly over an oven rack. Dry in 140°F oven until brittle (~4 hours). Note the time required. Store in a tightly closed container.

   b. *Unblanched, dry at 250°F (121°C)*—Prepare as in 2a, but dry at 250°F. Note the time required to become brittle. Store in a tightly sealed container.

   c. *Unblanched, dehydrator*—Prepare as in 2a, but dry in dehydrator at 140°F. Note the time required to become brittle. Store in a tightly sealed container.

3. **Drying of celery**—Wash each stalk thoroughly. Trim and slice into slices 1/4" thick. Divide the celery into 4 portions and use in the following methods.

   a. *Blanch, dry at 140°F (60°C)*—Place in basket and immerse in boiling water for 2 minutes. Drain and place on paper towels. Transfer to oven rack covered with cheesecloth; dry in 140°F oven until brittle (~4 hours).

   b. *Blanch, dry at 250°F (121°C)*—Prepare as in procedure 3a, but dry at 250°F.

   c. *Blanch, dehydrator, 140°F (60°C)*—Prepare as in procedure 3a, but dry in dehydrator at 140°F until brittle. Note time required.

   d. *Unblanched, dehydrator, 140°F (60°C)*—Prepare as in procedure 3a, but do not blanch. Dry in dehydrator at 140°F until brittle.

4. **Drying apples (or fresh peaches or grapes)**—Wash, core, and pare fruit (cut grapes in half). Cut into slices 1/8" thick. Use 1 apple for each variation.

   a. *Unblanched, ascorbic acid, 140°F (60°C)*—Dissolve 1/8 tsp ascorbic acid in 1/2 c water. Stir the apple slices into this solution. Drain slices thoroughly. Place on a cheesecloth-covered rack in an oven at 140°F. Note the time required to dry the slices.

   b. *Unblanched, no ascorbic acid, 140°F (60°C)*—Prepare as in procedure 4a, but omit the ascorbic acid rinse. Note the time required for drying.

   c. *Unblanched, ascorbic acid, 250°F (121°C)*—Prepare as in 4a, but dry in a 250°F oven. Note the time required for drying.

   d. *Unblanched, no ascorbic acid, 250°F (121°C)*—Prepare as in 4b (no ascorbic acid solution), but dry at 250°F. Note the time required for drying.

   e. *Unblanched, ascorbic acid, dehydrator at 140°F (60°C)*—Prepare as in 4a, but dry in a dehydrator at 140°F (60°C). Note the time required to dry.

   f. *Unblanched, no ascorbic acid, dehydrator at 140°F (60°C)*—Prepare as in 4b (no ascorbic acid solution), but dry in a dehydrator at 140°F. Note the time required to dry.

   g. *Blanched, ascorbic acid, 140°F (60°C)*—Prepare as in 4a, but blanch the slices for 2 minutes and blot dry with paper towels before placing slices in the ascorbic acid solution. Dry on cheesecloth-covered oven rack in a 140°F oven. Note the time required to dry.

   h. *Blanched, no ascorbic acid, 140°F (60°C)*—Prepare as in 4b, but blanch the slices for 2 minutes and blot dry with paper towels before drying (omit ascorbic acid solution). Dry on cheesecloth-covered rack in a 140°F oven. Note the time required to dry.

   i. *Blanched, ascorbic acid, 250°F (121°C)*—Prepare as in 4a, but blanch for 2 minutes and blot dry with paper towels before placing slices in the ascorbic acid solution. Dry on a cheesecloth-covered rack in a 250°F oven. Note the time required to dry.

j. *Blanched, no ascorbic acid, dehydrator at 140°F (60°C)*—Prepare as in 4b, but blanch for 2 minutes and dry on paper towels (omit ascorbic acid solution) before drying in a dehydrator at 140°F.

k. *Blanched, ascorbic acid, dehydrator*—Prepare as in procedure 4a, but blanch for 2 minutes and drain on paper towels before drying; dry in dehydrator at 140°F (60°C).

l. *Blanched, no ascorbic acid, dehydrator*—Prepare as in general procedure, but blanch for 2 minutes and drain on paper towels before drying; dry in dehydrator at 140°F (60°C).

BASIC FORMULA—FRUIT LEATHER

2 1/2 c	Strawberries, hulled and cut in half
25 g	Sugar

Puree strawberries in blender until smooth. Stir in the sugar. Line jelly roll pan with aluminum foil and fasten it to the edges with masking tape. Spread the fruit evenly in the pan. Dry in oven at 140°F (60°C) until completely dry and no longer sticky (approximately 12 hours). Remove from aluminum foil and roll up. Wrap the roll tightly in aluminum foil and store at room temperature in a tightly closed plastic bag or container. **Note:** Apple leather can be made using 1 1/2 lb of apples (peeled, cored, and pureed), 90 ml water, 75 g sugar, and 0.8 g cinnamon.

---

5. Fruit leather

a. *Control*—Prepare the basic formula. Note the time required to dry.

b. *Dehydrator*—Prepare basic formula, but place the pan in a dehydrator at 140°F (60°C). Note the time required to dry.

c. *Honey, 140°F (60°C) oven*—Prepare basic formula, but substitute 30 ml honey for the sugar. Dry in oven at 140°F. Note the time required to dry.

d. *Honey, dehydrator*—Prepare as in 5c, but place in a dehydrator at 140°F (60°C). Note the time required to dry.

EVALUATION

1. Allow dried onions to remain in storage at least 2 weeks before evaluating. Compare the cost of onions dried at home with the dried onions in the market. Sample a small amount of the home-dried product and compare it with the commercial product. Note any differences in color, texture, or flavor.

2. Evaluate parsley in the same manner as described for onions.

3. Drop celery into rapidly boiling water and boil 1 minute before tasting it. Note the texture, appearance, and flavor of the rehydrated dried product.

4. Evaluate apples in the same manner as described in evaluation 1 (onions). Note particularly any color, flavor, or textural differences resulting from the different drying techniques. Compare each variation with apples that have been dried commercially.

5. Compare the color of the leathers to determine whether there are differences caused by the sweeteners and/or by the drying method. Compare the flavor and tenderness, too.

STUDY QUESTIONS

1. Outline the basic method(s) for drying fruits and vegetables. What points need to be watched particularly when drying foods at home?

2. Why are some vegetables blanched? Are there some vegetables that are reduced in quality if they are blanched prior to being dried?

3. Should fruits be blanched before being dried? Why?

4. How does ascorbic acid function in the drying of apples?

5. Can any foods be dried satisfactorily at 250°F (121°C)? If so, which ones? Can other foods be dried at this high a temperature?

6. Compare the quality, convenience, and cost of home-dried and commercially dried vegetables and fruits. Which would you buy? Why?

CHART 12.2.1   DRIED VEGETABLES

Treatment	Home dried				Commercial	
	Color	**Flavor**	**Texture**	**Cost**	**Description**	**Cost**
1. Onion a. Blanched 140°F						
b. Unblanched, 140°F (control)						
c. Unblanched, 250°F						
d. Unblanched, dehydrator						
2. Parsley a. Unblanched, 140°F (control)						
b. Unblanched, 250°F						
c. Unblanched, dehydrator						
3. Celery a. Blanch, 140°F (control)						
b. Blanch, 250°F						
c. Blanch, dehydrator						
d. Unblanched, 140°F						

Name

ADDITIONAL OBSERVATIONS AND NOTES

CHART 12.2.2   DRIED FRUITS

Treatment	Home dried				Commercial	
	Color	**Flavor**	**Texture**	**Cost**	**Description**	**Cost**
4. Apples						
a. Unblanched asc. ac., 140°F (control)						
b. Unblanched, no asc. ac., 140°F						
c. Unblanched, asc. ac., 250°F						
d. Unblanched, no asc. ac., 250°F						
e. Unblanched, asc. ac., dehydr.						
f. Unblanched, no asc. ac., dehydr.						
g. Blanched, asc. ac., 140°F						
h. Blanched, no asc. ac., 140°F						
i. Blanched, asc. ac., 250°F						
j. Blanched, no asc. ac., 250°F						
k. Blanched, asc. ac., dehydr.						
l. Blanched, no asc. ac., dehydr.						

Name

ADDITIONAL OBSERVATIONS AND NOTES

Chart 12.2.3   Fruit Leathers

Treatment	Color	Flavor	Tenderness	Texture
a. Sugar, 140°F (control)				
b. Sugar, dehydrator				
c. Honey, 140°F				
d. Honey, dehydrator				

Name

ADDITIONAL OBSERVATIONS AND NOTES

EXPERIMENT 12.3—JELLY
OBJECTIVES

Upon completion of the experiment, you will be able to:

1. Explain the role of each of the following in the formation of pectin gels: pectin, acid, and sugar.
2. Outline the changes in yield, appearance, and tenderness that occur in jellies as temperature, sugar content, pH, and level of pectin are varied.
3. Explain and perform the objective tests used for evaluating tenderness of gels.

BASIC FORMULA—JELLY

1.36 kg (3 lb)	Tart apples
708 ml (3c)	Water*
30 ml (2 tbsp)	Lemon juice
600 g (3 c)	Sugar

*Note: Water and apples to yield 944 ml extracted juice.

Pectin extraction—Select apples that are a mixture of underripe and fully ripe tart apples. Wash thoroughly and cut away bruises and other imperfections; remove the blossom end and the stem. Cut the remaining apple (including skin, seeds, and core) into small pieces. Place the water and apples in a large kettle. Cover and heat quickly to boiling. Reduce heat to maintain a simmering temperature for 20 to 25 minutes, until apples are tender. Dampen a jelly bag or double layer of cheesecloth stretched over a colander. Place bag over a container to collect the material extracted from the apples. Let juice drip through the bag without pressing. If there is not enough juice, remove the original collection of clear juice, and place another container under the bag to collect the additional juice that is released by gently squeezing the bag. Filter this second collection through fresh cheesecloth to help clarify it before using it. This procedure extracts pectin from the fruit (primarily from the seeds and core). Measure 944 ml of juice for use in the jelly experiment. Reserve any additional extracted juice for use by other groups, if needed.

Method for jelly—Pour 944 ml of extracted apple juice into a 3-quart saucepan. Add the lemon juice and sugar. Stir well to help dissolve the sugar while heating rapidly to a boil. Boil rapidly until the thermometer indicates 4.4C° (8F°) above the boiling point of water in the laboratory. Immediately remove from the heat, skim off the foam with a slotted spoon, and pour into jelly glasses that have been washed and rinsed in scalding water. Seal with a layer of paraffin ~ 1/8" thick. Pop any bubbles that form in the paraffin.

PROCEDURE

1. **Jellies boiled to different temperatures**—This series is to be done by one group.

   a. *Boiling point 2.2 C° (4 F°) above boiling water*—Prepare basic formula as outlined above, but very carefully remove enough of the jelly to fill a glass 3/4 full when the temperature is 2.2 C° above the boiling point of water.

b. *Boiling point 4.4 C° (8 F°) above boiling point of water (control)*—Continue to boil the jelly remaining in the kettle after removing sample 1a. Remove a similar sample when the temperature rises to 4.4 C° above the boiling point of water. Determine the pH of the jelly.

c. *Boiling point 6.6 C° (12 F°) above boiling point of water*—Continue to boil the remaining jelly until the temperature rises to 6.6 C° (12 F°) above the boiling point of water. Pour the remaining jelly into 1 or more glasses.

2. **Jellies with varying levels of sugar**—Prepare a batch of pectin extract from 3 lb of apples, as outlined above. Use 236 ml of extracted juice for each of the following variations and 7 1/2 ml lemon juice plus the amount of sugar indicated. Boil to 4.4 C° (8 F°) above the boiling point of water. Immediately pour all of the jelly into glasses. Add paraffin layer, as described in the basic formula. (**Note:** Pectin extract is to be prepared by one group and shared with the others making this series.)

   a. *100 g sugar*—Prepare jelly as outlined in procedure 2; use 100 g sugar.

   b. *125 g sugar*—Prepare jelly as outlined in procedure 2; use 125 g sugar.

   c. *175 g sugar*—Prepare jelly as outlined in procedure 2; use 175 g sugar.

   d. *200 g sugar*—Prepare jelly as outlined in procedure 2; use 200 g sugar.

3. **Jellies with varying levels of acid**—Prepare a batch of pectin extract from 3 lb of apples, as outlined in the basic formula. Use 472 ml of the extracted juice and 300 g sugar for each of the variations. Vary the lemon juice as indicated. Boil to 4.4 C° (8 F°) above the boiling point of water. Immediately pour all of the jelly into glasses and add paraffin layer. (**Note:** Pectin extract is to be made by one group and shared with the other.)

   a. *0 ml lemon juice*—Prepare jelly as outlined in procedure 3, but add no lemon juice. Determine the pH of the mixture.

   b. *30 ml lemon juice*—Prepare jelly as outlined in procedure 3, but add 30 ml lemon juice. Determine the pH of the mixture.

4. **Jellies with varying levels and types of pectin**

   a. *Control*—Prepare jelly as described in the basic formula. Determine the pH of the mixture after cooking.

   b. *Powdered pectin, 1/2 recommendation*—Prepare half the basic formula (236 ml juice and 350 g sugar). Measure juice, as described in the basic formula. To the juice, add 1/8 package of powdered pectin (weigh total package and then weigh out exactly 1/8 of the total weight of powdered pectin). Bring the juice and pectin to a full boil, stirring constantly. Add sugar and boil hard 1 minute. Skim off foam with a slotted spoon before pouring into jelly glasses and adding paraffin, as described in the basic formula.

   c. *Powdered pectin, recommended pectin level*—Place 236 ml juice and 1/4 package (by weight) of powdered pectin in a saucepan. Heat quickly to a rolling boil, stirring constantly. Add 350 g sugar and boil hard 1 minute. Skim off foam with a slotted spoon before pouring into jelly glasses and adding paraffin (see basic formula).

d. *Powdered pectin, 1 1/2x recommendation*—Place 236 ml juice and 3/8 package (by weight) of powdered pectin in a saucepan. Heat quickly to a rolling boil, stirring constantly. Add 350 g sugar and boil hard 1 minute. Remove from heat, skim off the foam with a slotted spoon before pouring into jelly glasses and adding paraffin (see basic formula).

EVALUATION

Objective evaluation   If a penetrometer is available, measure tenderness of the gel using it. If a penetrometer is not available, tenderness can be measured by determining the percent sag. This test requires that the height of the molded jelly be measured by inserting a skewer downward until its point touches the glass at the bottom of the jelly. This distance is measured when the skewer is withdrawn. After the jelly is carefully unmolded onto a plate, the height of the unmolded jelly at its center is again measured. The percent (%) sag is determined by the following calculation:

$$\% \text{ sag} = \frac{\text{molded height} - \text{unmolded height}}{\text{molded height}} \times 100$$

Yield of jellies is important. The yield of each variation can be determined by marking the height of the jelly on the exterior of each glass before the jelly is unmolded. After the jelly is unmolded, the glass is filled with water to the mark, and the volume of the water is measured in a graduated cylinder.

Subjective evaluation   Unmold all of the jellies onto plates for subjective evaluation. Jellies should be evaluated subjectively for color, clarity, flavor, tenderness, and syneresis.

STUDY QUESTIONS

1. What are the three essential ingredients in any jelly? What is the role performed by each? Explain the roles in relation to a commonly accepted theory of gel formation.

2. What effects are noted when the content of sugar is increased? When pectin is increased? When acid is increased?

3. Describe the process used for extracting pectin from fruits.

4. Describe the process for adding liquid pectin to jellies; for adding powdered pectin.

5. What effect does final temperature have on jellies? Why is temperature an indication of when jelly is done?

6. Explain the method for determining percent sag. If a reading for percent sag is higher for one jelly than for another, which jelly is more tender?

CHART 12.3   JELLIES

Treatment	Objective			Subjective				
	Tenderness % sag or pene.	pH	Vol. (ml)	Color	Clarity	Flavor	Tenderness	Syneresis
1. Boil a. +2.2°C			XXX					
b. +4.4°C, control								
c. +6.6°C			XXX					
2. Sugar a. 100 g			XXX					
b. 125 g			XXX					
150 g, control (see 1b)			XXX					
c. 175 g			XXX					
d. 200 g			XXX					
3. Acid a. 0 ml								
15 ml, control (see 1b)								
b. 30 ml								
4. Pectin a. Liquid pectin								
b. Powd., 1/2 pectin			XXX					
c. Powd., 1 pectin			XXX					
d. Powd., 1 1/2 pectin			XXX					

Name

ADDITIONAL OBSERVATIONS AND NOTES

Appendix A
Basic Techniques

PREPARING SAMPLES

Meaningful results in an experimental foods laboratory can be obtained only when all participants work carefully and use standardized procedures to eliminate as many human variables as possible. Ingredients, except for the liquids, are weighed on a laboratory balance; liquids are measured in graduated cylinders. Measures are in the metric system, the system used in science laboratories (Appendix B).

USE OF BALANCES

Weighing ingredients will seem cumbersome and time consuming at first, but the accuracy achieved through the use of balances more than compensates for the inconvenience. Attention should be given in the laboratory toward developing the skill required for relatively rapid weighing of ingredients. Directions for using the trip balance, triple beam balance, and the torsion balance are presented below. Manufacturer's directions should be followed for using other types of balances that may be available in the laboratory.

Operating the Trip Balance

1. Remove the rubber ring locks. Place the rider weight on 0.

2. Balance the needle to 0 by using the adjustment screws.

3. If the balance does not move readily, check to see if the indicating needle is bent or if food has been spilled in any part of the balance. Make any necessary adjustments so that it moves freely.

4. Place comparable containers on both pans of the balance. These may simply be matching pieces of paper for holding the food to be weighed, matching measuring cups, plastic containers, or other suitable devices for holding food.

5. Check to see if the needle still indicates 0. If not, be sure that the lighter container is on the *right* pan.

6. Add paper, water, or shot (whichever is most convenient) in the container on the *right* pan of the balance until the balance needle is at 0.

7. Using the rider on the balance or weights (transferred to the *right* pan by tweezers), add the weight indicated in the experiment for the ingredient being weighed.

8. Add the ingredient to the container on the *left* pan until the balance needle indicates 0. This completes the weighing.

9. Return the rider on the balance to 0, and remove any weights that have been used.

10. Subsequent weighings can be done most efficiently if the balance remains in its original position on the counter so that it is not necessary to readjust the balance to 0. If moved, possible variations in the counter surface make it necessary to readjust the balance so that the needle points to 0.

11. For subsequent weighings, repeat steps 4 through 9.

Operating the Triple Beam Balance

The triple beam balance is operated as follows:

1. Place all riders on 0, and remove the support from under the pan.

2. Balance the needle to 0 by using the adjustment screws.

3. Put the support beneath the pan to hold it while moving the rider(s) to the desired weight(s) on the beams.

4. Remove the support and begin to add the ingredient gradually, continuing until the needle indicates 0.

5. Be sure the pan is perfectly clean and dry before returning it to the balance for subsequent weighings.

Using the Torsion Balance

The torsion balance is operated as follows:

1. Observe the location of the bubble in the circle. If the bubble is not centered, adjust the legs of the balance to center it.

2. Gently release the lever that locks the pans. Note whether the pans seem to be able to move up and down freely. If not, find the cause of the friction and correct the problem after locking the pans in position.

3. Release the pans again and observe whether the needle points to 0. If not, turn the adjustment screws to bring it to 0.

4. Lock the pans in position.

5. Add containers of equal weight on each pan, as described for the trip balance in step 4.

6. Release the pans to see whether the needle still points to 0. If not, put the lighter container on the right.

7. With the pans released, carefully add paper, water, or shot to the right side to bring the needle to 0.

8. Lock the pans.

9. Add the weight desired for the ingredient to be weighed by using the rider and/or appropriate weights (added using tweezers).

10. Carefully release the pans.

11. Add the ingredient to the container on the left gradually until the needle indicates 0.

12. Lock the pans and remove the weighed ingredient.

13. Subsequent weighings are done using the same technique, being careful to avoid shifting the position of the balance at all.

EXERCISES

1. Use a trip balance to weigh 105 grams of shortening.

2. Use a triple beam balance to weigh 4 grams of salt.

3. Use a torsion balance to weigh 330 grams of flour.

STUDY QUESTIONS

1. Outline the steps to follow in using a trip balance.

2. How should a trip balance be stored?

3. Outline the steps to follow in using a triple beam balance.

4. How should a triple beam balance be stored?

5. Outline the steps to follow in using a torsion balance.

6. How should a torsion balance be stored?

EXPERIMENT A.1—ACCURACY OF HOME MEASURES
OBJECTIVES

Upon completion of the experiment, you will be able to:

1. Contrast the accuracy of home measuring equipment and weighing ingredients on a balance.
2. Discuss the merits of sifting flour when flour is weighed.
3. Identify the problems associated with measuring solid fats and brown sugar using home measuring equipment.
4. Compare the accuracy of volume measurements using a home measuring cup and a graduated cylinder.

7. Which type of balance is best suited to weighing each of the following: (a) 110 g flour, (b) 50 g sugar, (c) 1 g baking powder, and (d) 0.5 g cinnamon?

PROCEDURE

1. Weigh the assigned variation 3 times; record the results in Chart A.1. Calculate the means.

   a. *All purpose flour sifted and spooned*—Sift all purpose flour once and then lightly spoon it into the graduated measuring cup until very full. Scrape level using the straight side of a metal spatula. Weigh each of the following measures:

   1 cup

   1/2 cup

   1/4 cup

   b. *All purpose flour unsifted and spooned*—Spoon unsifted all purpose flour into the graduated measuring cup until very full. Scrape level using the straight side of a metal spatula. Weigh each of the following measures:

   1 cup

   1/2 cup

   1/4 cup

   c. *All purpose flour sifted into measuring cup*—Sift all purpose flour directly into the graduated measuring cup until very full. Scrape level using the straight side of a metal spatula. Weigh each of the following measures:

   1 cup

   1/2 cup

   1/4 cup

d. *Hydrogenated shortening*—Press hydrogenated shortening firmly into the graduated measuring cup. Scrape level using the straight edge of a metal spatula. Weigh each of the following measures:

1 cup

1/2 cup

1/4 cup

e. *Brown sugar, pressed*—Press brown sugar gently into the graduated measuring cup. Scrape level using the straight edge of a metal spatula. Weigh each of the following measures:

1 cup

1/2 cup

1/4 cup

f. *Brown sugar, spooned*—Repeat 1e, but spoon sugar without pressing.

1 cup

1/2 cup

1/4 cup

2. Weigh the following measures (leveled with a metal spatula) of baking soda, and record the results in Chart A.1:

1 tablespoon

1 teaspoon

1/2 teaspoon

1/4 teaspoon

3. Fill a glass measuring cup to the following levels, and then pour the water into a graduated cylinder. Be sure to read the bottom of the meniscus in each measurement. Record the results in Chart A.1.

1 cup

3/4 cup

2/3 cup

1/2 cup

1/3 cup

1/4 cup

STUDY QUESTIONS

1. Using the results recorded in Chart A.1, identify the most accurate home measuring technique for measuring (a) all purpose flour and (b) brown sugar.

2. Which is more accurate for measuring dry ingredients: using a balance or using the most accurate home measuring technique?

3. Is it necessary to sift all purpose flour before weighing? Explain your answer.

4. Using the values obtained by sifting and spooning flour into various graduated measuring cups, answer the following comparisons. Was the weight of 1 cup of flour equal to (a) two times the weight of 1/2 cup of flour, (b) four times the weight of 1/4 cup of flour? Explain.

5. Compare the mean value of the weight of 1 cup of shortening with (a) 4 times the mean weight of 1/4 cup of shortening and (b) 2 times the mean weight of 1/2 cup. Are these values the same? Why?

6. Compare the weight of a tablespoon of baking soda with each of the following: (a) 3 times the weight of 1 teaspoon, (b) 6 times the weight of 1/2 teaspoon, (c) 12 times the weight of 1/4 teaspoon. How does this information influence how small amounts of dry ingredients can be measured most accurately in the laboratory and in the home? Explain.

7. Compare the actual volumes in the graduated cylinder with the expected volumes of water. Explain the reason for the discrepancies.

CHART A.1   ACCURACY OF HOME MEASURES

Treatment	Weight in grams					
	1 cup		1/2 cup		1/4 cup	
	Individual	Mean	Individual	Mean	Individual	Mean
1. Large measures a. All purpose flour, sifted						
b. All purpose flour, unsifted						
c. All purpose flour, sifted in cup						
d. Shortening						
e. Brown sugar, pressed						
f. Brown sugar, spooned						

Measurement	(g)	(ml)
2. Soda a. 1 tablespoon		XXX
b. 1 teaspoon		XXX
c. 1/2 teaspoon		XXX
d. 1/4 teaspoon		XXX
3. Water a. 1 cup	XXX	
b. 3/4 cup	XXX	
c. 2/3 cup	XXX	
d. 1/2 cup	XXX	
e. 1/3 cup	XXX	
f. 1/4 cup	XXX	

Name

ADDITIONAL OBSERVATIONS AND NOTES

EVALUATION

Subjective Testing

Although class work is, of necessity, somewhat crowded physically and time is limited, it still is possible to create the environment needed to begin to develop evaluation skills. The products of experiments should be labeled carefully and arranged for scoring in a meaningful display for all to see. Where appropriate, exterior evaluation of products should be conducted before cutting into individual samples.

Students need to mark their sample plates carefully with wax pencil so that samples can be identified when evaluation is being done in a quiet part of the laboratory. Ideally, evaluation is done in a tasting booth.

Evaluation is best done individually, with the notes and comments being recorded on the charts for the experiments. Careful comparison of experimental variations will reveal important aspects of food science. The ability to evaluate food accurately will develop gradually as careful examination and a questioning mind are used in analyzing samples in the laboratory.

Objective Testing

Objective testing can provide important information about such significant characteristics as volume, tenderness, flow properties, gel strength, and emulsion stability if the necessary equipment is available. However, it is essential that objective testing equipment be maintained well and that tests are done using the equipment correctly and carefully. Objective testing equipment available in the laboratory differs considerably. Operation of equipment that often is available in student laboratories is described in this section.

VOLUMETER AND ITS OPERATION

Volume is a key characteristic in evaluating the quality of breads, cakes, and other baked products. Seed displacement is the technique commonly used to measure volume; water displacement can used, but is inconvenient because of the problem of separating the food from the water. A volumeter can be used to measure volume by seed displacement. The steps in its operation are as follows:

1. With the grate open in the column, fill the volumeter by pouring rape seeds into the top of the column slowly until the seeds can be measured near the lower end of the visible calibrated column. Record the initial reading.

2. Be sure the lid has been replaced and locked on at the top of the volumeter. With the grate still open in the column, rotate the volumeter down so that the upper compartment is lowered sufficiently to cause almost all of the seeds to fall into that compartment.

3. Close the grate in the column to trap the seeds before rotating the volumeter to its upright position.

4. Double check to be sure that almost all of the seeds are trapped in the upper compartment and that the lid on that compartment is locked securely. Then unlock the lower compartment and insert the sample in it. Lock the sample box.

5. Check to be sure the lower compartment with the sample is locked, and then quickly slide the grate plate into the column so the seeds can fall into the sample box, surrounding the sample and rising upward in the visible column until all of the seeds have fallen. Record this final volume.

6. To remove the sample, check to be sure that both compartments are locked securely. Then rotate the volumeter to shift the seeds back into the upper compartment.

7. While the upper compartment is still in the downward position, slide the grate out of the column. This blocks the seeds in the upper compartment.

8. Rotate the volumeter back to its original position. Check to be sure that the upper compartment is filled with the seeds before unlocking the lower compartment and removing the sample.

9. Calculate the volume of the sample using the equation:

$$\text{final volume} - \text{initial volume} = \text{volume of sample}$$

SHORTOMETER AND ITS OPERATION

Tenderness of crisp baked products such as pastry, crackers, and thin cookies can be measured objectively using a shortometer. The thickness of samples must be controlled so that scores of various samples can be compared. To help eliminate variability between specific samples, it is wise to test three or more samples from the same experimental variation. The mean of the values can be compared with the mean of values obtained testing other experimental variations if each of the samples is the same thickness. The smaller the reading obtained on the shortometer, the more tender the product being tested. This usually is the desired characteristic. It is important to remember that the food with the lowest score is usually the most tender.

Operation of the shortometer is done as follows:

1. Check to be sure that the indicator (rider) needle is positioned in front of the pressure gauge.

2. Release the pressure bar if it is not already in its resting position well above the sample bars.

3. Place the sample across the sample bars so that it extends about the same distance beyond the parallel bars.

4. Press the button to lower the pressure bar and continue pressing until the sample snaps.

5. Record the pressure marked by the rider, which remains in its position at the time of the break. (The pressure gauge needle springs back to its earlier position as soon as the sample breaks and does not indicate the maximum pressure reached.)

SHEAR AND ITS OPERATION

The shear can be used to measure relative tenderness of meat, cookies with a chewy texture, and other foods that afford enough resistance to the shearing force to provide a reading on the gauge before they tear apart. The higher the reading, the less tender the sample being tested. Results from shearing samples of identical dimensions and from comparable location on a meat carcass can be compared to determine relative tenderness. The relative tenderness of other foods capable of being measured on the shear can also be determined if samples being tested are prepared carefully to be as similar as possible.

The shear is operated as follows:

1. Be sure the needle of the rider on the dial is situated in front of the pressure gauge.

2. Cut the sample to controlled dimensions (preferably cut using a coring device that will cut a cylindrical sample that can be inserted through the aperture in the shear).

3. Adjust the shear so that the shearing bars are above the aperture for the sample before the sample is placed in position.

4. Holding the sample near one end of the core, insert it into the aperture far enough for the blades to shear the sample without contacting the fingers.

5. As soon as the bars begin to press against the sample, the gauge will begin to register the pressure being exerted against the food. When the sample is sheared apart, the pressure is relieved, and the gauge snaps back to 0, but the rider remains at the pressure point when shearing occurred.

6. Read the pressure indicated by the rider and record it. Return the rider to its correct position just in front of the pressure gauge.

PENETROMETER AND ITS OPERATION

The penetrometer is useful in measuring tenderness of jellies, custards, and foods with similar textures. The test measures the distance a testing device (e.g., a cone, needle, or other device of an appropriate weight and shape) travels downward into the sample when allowed to fall freely for a defined period of time. The higher the reading, the more tender the food.

Tests using the penetrometer are conducted as follows:

1. Check to be sure that the dial gauge is set at zero.

2. Pull up the rod attached to the cone or other testing device until it is in contact with the bar that is connected to the dial gauge.

3. Move this assembly high enough to permit the sample to be placed on the stand. Position the sample so that the testing device will enter the center of the sample.

4. Lower the assembly until the testing device barely contacts the surface of the sample. Tighten the adjustment knob to lock the assembly in this position.

5. Release the test device for a carefully defined period of time (determined by the length of time for the testing device to move part way through the sample without reaching the bottom). Relock the test device immediately when the specified number of seconds has elapsed.

6. Gently lower the handle attached to the dial gauge just until it contacts the top of the rod holding the testing device. The distance that the rod has moved indicates the tenderness of the gel. The **higher** the value, the **more tender** the product. Note that this is the reverse of the scores from the shear and shortometer tests, both of which indicate that products with **high** values are **less tender.**

LINE SPREAD TEST AND ITS CONDUCT

Flow properties of viscous liquids can be compared by conducting a line spread test. The equipment needed for this test includes a template of concentric circles (see Appendix D), a transparent plastic or glass sheet large enough to cover the pattern, and a short metal cylinder (a small biscuit cutter with the handle removed or some similar device).

The line spread test is conducted as follows.

1. Place the transparent sheet on the template and then position the metal cylinder to align with the center circle of the template.

2. Fill the cylinder (or to a defined level if too deep).

3. Lift the ring vertically and simultaneously begin timing elapsed time until readings are to be taken. (**Note:** A designated time appropriate to allow the sample to flow outward a measurable amount needs to be used for all samples in a single experiment so that comparisons can be made between samples.)

4. Immediately after the elapsed time, read the distance the sample has traveled at 4 discrete points separated by 90° from each other. The score is the mean of the 4 readings.

The thinner the viscous liquid being tested, the higher will be the mean score for the line spread test. Valid tests can be done only on samples that are (a) sufficiently viscous to flow only within the dimensions of the template and (b) sufficiently fluid to exhibit some measurable flow on the template. Samples that are too viscous for the line spread test probably can be tested using the penetrometer. Those samples that are too fluid for the line spread can be tested by using a burette to measure flow during a defined period.

PERCENT SAG AND ITS CONDUCT

Percent (%) sag is a convenient test for measuring gel strength and requires only a skewer and a centimeter ruler (see Appendix B). The stronger the gel, the smaller the % sag. Conversely, a large value for % sag indicates a very soft gel. [**Note:** The interpretation of the % sag scores (i.e., larger value means increasing tenderness and conversely, smaller value means decreasing tenderness) is comparable to interpretation of penetrometer scores for tenderness.]

The test for % sag is conducted as follows:

1. Before unmolding the sample, insert a skewer vertically in the center of the (molded) sample until the skewer contacts the bottom of the mold. Before removing the skewer, mark the height of the gel on the skewer.

2. Using a centimeter ruler, measure the height of the gel, as indicated on the skewer.

3. Carefully unmold the gel onto a flat plate.

4. Measure the height of the unmolded gel, using the measuring described in steps 1 and 2.

5. Calculate the % sag as follows:

$$\% \text{ sag} = \frac{\text{molded height} - \text{unmolded height}}{\text{molded height}} \times 100$$

CENTRIFUGE AND ITS OPERATION

A centrifuge is a useful device for determining relative stability of emulsions. The centrifugal force developed as the products spin gradually causes the heavier material to move toward the bottom of each tube.

A centrifuge is operated as follows:

1. Comparable amounts of sample are placed in matching centrifuge tubes and positioned opposite each other in the centrifuge.

2. The lid is placed on the centrifuge, and the machine is spun under controlled conditions of rate and time.

3. Before the lid is removed, the machine is turned off and allowed to coast to a stop without being touched.

4. Samples are checked after the lid is removed. Samples in which the emulsion has broken are removed.

5. If some samples have not yet separated, balance the centrifuge again by placing comparable samples opposite each other. The centrifuge always needs to be balanced with comparable loads opposite each other.

Appendix B
Essentials of the Metric System

PREFIXES

To operate with the metric system, it is necessary to know the prefixes used with the base units and their numeric definitions. The following presentation includes prefixes in the system, but kilo-, centi-, and milli- are the ones used most commonly in food experimentation.

Prefix (abbreviation)

tera	T	$10^{12} = 1,000,000,000,000$
giga	G	$10^9 = 1,000,000,000$
mega	M	$10^6 = 1,000,000$
kilo	K	$10^3 = 1,000$
hecto	H	$10^2 = 100$
deka	da	$10^1 = 10$
		$10^0 = 1$
deci	d	$10^{-1} = 0.1$
centi	c	$10^{-2} = 0.01$
milli	m	$10^{-3} = 0.001$
micro	μ	$10^{-6} = 0.000001$
nano	n	$10^{-9} = 0.000000001$

BASE UNITS AND EQUIVALENCIES

Mass and abbreviation

pound (lb) =	453.6 grams (g)
ounce (oz) =	28.35 grams (g)
kilogram (kg) =	2.21 pounds (lb)

343

Volume (abbreviation)

quart (qt) =	0.946 liter (l)
cup (c) =	236.6 milliliters (ml)
teaspoon (tsp) =	4.93 milliliters (ml)
tablespoon (tbsp) =	14.79 milliliters (ml)
fluid ounce (fl oz) =	29.57 milliliters (ml)
liter (l) =	1.057 quarts (qt)

Length (abbreviation)

inch (in)	2.54 centimeters (cm)
yard (yd)	0.914 meter (m)
meter (m)	39.37 inches (in)

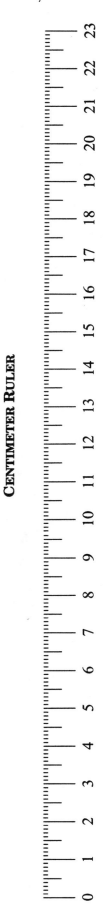

Appendix C
Temperature Conversions

°F (left scale)		°C (right scale)
220°F		
	212°F — BOILING POINT OF WATER	100°C
210°F		
200°F		
	194°F	90°C
190°F		
180°F	176°F	80°C
170°F		
160°F	158°F	70°C
150°F		
140°F	140°F	60°C
130°F		
120°F	122°F	50°C
110°F		
100°F	104°F	40°C
90°F	86°F	30°C
80°F		
70°F	68°F	20°C
60°F		
50°F	50°F	10°C
40°F		
30°F	32°F — FREEZING POINT OF WATER	0°C
20°F		
10°F	14°F	-10°C
0°F		

TEMPERATURE CONVERSIONS

$$°C = (°F - 32) \times 5/9$$

$$°F = (°C \times 9/5) + 32$$

Appendix D
Template for Line Spread Test

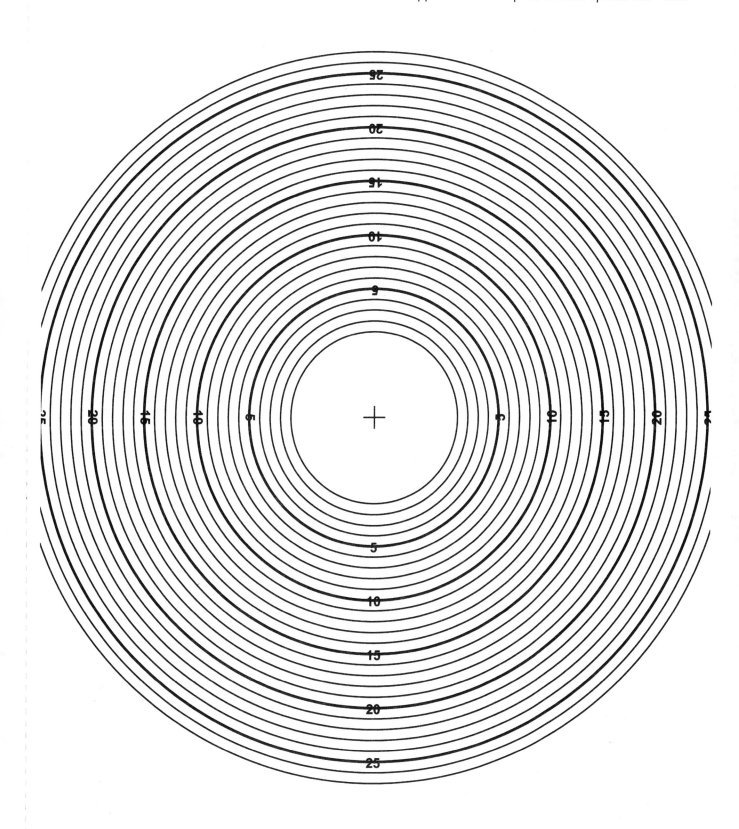

Appendix E

Average Weight of a Measured Cup of Selected Foods

AVERAGE WEIGHT OF A MEASURED CUP OF SELECTED FOODS[a]

Food	Form	Weight (g/c)	Food	Form	Weight (g/c)
Almonds	Blanched, whole	157	great northern	Dry, uncooked	178
	Blanched, chopped	127	green	Fresh, uncooked	107
Apples	Raw, pared		mung	Dry, uncooked	203
	chopped	124	pea	Dry, uncooked	199
	diced	109	soy	Dry, uncooked	173
	quartered	122	tofu	Curd, 1/2" cubes	184
	sliced	108	Beef, ground	Uncooked	226
	Cooked, sliced, no sugar	207	Bread	Crumbs, dry	107
				Crumbs, soft	43
Baking powder	Double acting	177		Cubes, dry	42
				Cubes, soft	40
Barley	Uncooked	195	Bulgur	Uncooked	140
Beans			Cheese		
black	Dry, uncooked	184	cheddar	Shredded	98

355

Food	Form	Weight (g/c)	Food	Form	Weight (g/c)
cottage	Creamed	233		White, unsifted	149
cream	Original	230	rye	Dark, stirred	127
mozzarella	Chopped	112		Light, unsifted	101
Swiss	Shredded	108		Whole-grain, unsifted	82
Chicken	Cooked, deboned	144	soy	Full-fat, unsifted	96
Chocolate	Chips	167	tapioca	Unsifted	120
Cocoa		86	wheat	All purpose	
Cocoa mix		139		unsifted, spooned	126
Coconut				unsifted, dipped	143
fresh	Grated	80		sifted, spooned	116
dried	Flakes	88		Bread	
dried	Shredded	91		unsifted, spooned	123
Cookies				unsifted, dipped	136
gingersnaps	Crumbs	115		sifted, spooned	117
vanilla wafers	Crumbs	104		Cake	
Corn grits	Uncooked	162		unsifted, spooned	111
Cornmeal				unsifted, dipped	119
white	Uncooked	140		sifted, spooned	99
yellow	Uncooked	151		Gluten	
Corn syrup		325		unsifted, spooned	135
Crackers				unsifted, dipped	142
graham	Crumbs	84		sifted, spooned	136
snack	Crumbs	80		Self-rising	
Cream				unsifted, spooned	127
sour		242		unsifted, dipped	130
whipping		232		sifted, spooned	106
Currants	Dehydrated	131		Whole wheat	
Dates	Dehydrated, pitted, chopped	171		stirred, spooned	120
			Gelatin	Flavored	187
Eggs			Honey	Strained	325
whites		255	Lemon	Juice	223
whole		251	Lemon	Fresh juice	250
yolks		240	Lentils	Dry, uncooked	186
Flour			Macaroni	Elbow, uncooked	130
barley	Unsifted, spooned	102	Margarine	Regular	225
oat	Coarse, unsifted	120		Soft	208
	Fine, unsifted	96	Milk	Fresh, fluid	
potato	Unsifted, spooned	179		whole	241
rice	Brown, unsifted	158		skim	246

Food	Form	Weight (g/c)	Food	Form	Weight (g/c)
	Nonfat, dry	74	Rice		
	instant	134	brown	Long grain, raw	176
	spray	124		Short grain, raw	194
Molasses		309	white	Long grain, raw	192
Mustard	Prepared	251		Short grain, raw	200
Noodles	Uncooked, medium	38		Parboiled, raw	181
	Uncooked, thin	45	Mayonnaise	Regular	240
Oats, rolled	Quick, uncooked	73	Sugar	Brown, packed	211
	Regular, uncooked	75		Brownulated	152
Oil	Cooking	209		Confectioner's, unsifted	113
Onions, dry	Uncooked			Confectioner's, sifted	95
	chopped	171		Granulated	196
	grated	231		Raw, pared	195
	ground	238		Superfine	197
	slices	113	Sunflower	Seeds, hulled	125
Parsley	Dried, flakes	15	Tapioca	Quick-cooking	160
Peanut butter	Crunchy	261	Walnuts	English, chopped	120
	Smooth	251	Wheat	Germ, spooned	115
Peanuts	Salted, chopped	138		Starch, unsifted, spooned	123
Pecans, shelled	Chopped	108	Whey	Liquid	244
	Halves	108	Yeast	Active dry	142
Potatoes	Fresh, raw, diced	161	Yogurt	Whole milk	245
	Dry flakes	55		Partially skimmed	249
	Dry granules	201			
Raisins	Uncooked, whole	144			

Appendix F
Examples of Bibliographic Styles

The bibliography is part of reporting research projects. Citations can be reported in a variety of ways. When writing a paper to submit to a specific journal, it is necessary to follow the style used in that journal. Check the journal to find its style guide for authors. In the absence of specific guidelines for writing the bibliography, it is acceptable to follow the style used in an appropriate professional journal. Some of the journals appropriate for food researchers include *Food Technology, Journal of Food Science,* and the *Journal of the American Dietetic Association.* Some examples of the styles used in these journals are presented below to aid in writing a bibliography for a research paper written for this course. Particular attention should be paid to the punctuation and capitalization used in the style selected for preparing the bibliography. It is important to be consistent in the format used for all entries. Use one appropriate model and follow it for each bibliographic entry.

EXAMPLES FROM *FOOD TECHNOLOGY*

Book

Brody, A. L. and Lord, J. 2000. "Developing New Food Products for a Changing Marketplace." CRC Press, Boca Raton, Fla.

Periodical Article

Booth, S. L., Broe, K. E., Gagnon, D. R., Tucker, K. L, Hannon, M. T., McLean, R. R., Dawson-Hughes, B., Wilson, P. W. F., Cupples, L./A., and Kiel, D. P. 2003. Vitamin K intake and bone mineral density in women and men. Am. J. Clin. Nutr. 77:512–516.

Citation from a Compilation

Tannock, G. W. 1999. Intestinal microflora. In "Probiotics: Critical Review," ed. G. W. Tannock. Pp. 5–14. Horizon Scientific Press, Norfolk, England.

Thesis

Wong, P. J. 1999. Comparison of alternative sweeteners in shortened cakes. M.S. thesis. Ultima University, Woodbridge, NM.

Internet

IRI. 2002. What do Americans really eat survey? Information Resources, Inc. Chicago. www.infores.com

EXAMPLES FROM *JOURNAL OF FOOD SCIENCE*

Book

Preis J. 1999. The biochemistry of plants. San Diego: Academic Press. 450 p.

Citation in a Compilation

Furda J. 1990. Interaction of dietary fiber with lipids—mechanistic theories and their limitations. In: Furda I., Brine C. J., editors. Advances in experimental medicine and biology. New York: Plenum Press. p. 67–82.

Periodical Article

Gutema T., Muniumbazi C., Bullerman L. K. B. 2000. Occurrence of fumonisuns and moniliformin in corn and corn-based food products of U.S. origin. J Food Prot 63(12): 1732–7.

Dissertation

Castelo M. 1999. Stability of mycotoxins in thermally processed corn products. [dissertation] Lincoln, NE: Univ. of Nebraska-Lincoln. p. 77–92.

EXAMPLES FROM *JOURNAL OF THE AMERICAN DIETETIC ASSOCIATION*

Book

Rolinick S., Mason P., Butler C. *Health Behavior Change: A Guide for Practitioners.* New York, NY: Churchill Livingstone. 1999.

Periodical Article

Slavin J., Jacobs D., Marquart L., Wiemer K. The role of whole grains in disease prevention. *J Am Diet Assoc 2001; 101:*780–785.

Internet

Environmental Protection Agency. MSW Management Basic Fact. Available at http:www.epa.gov/epaoswer/non-hw/muncpl/fact.htm. Accessed February 13, 2003.

Dissertation

Wie S. *Cost Analysis of Alternative Disposal Methods for Wastes Generated by Foodservice Operations* [dissertation]. Manhattan, KS: Kansas State University. 2000.

Citation from a Compilation

Patterson R. E. Preview of Nutritional Epidemiology. In: Coulston M., Rock C. L, Monsen E., eds. *Nutrition in the Prevention and Treatment of Disease.* San Diego, CA: Academic Press; 2001.

Government Publication

U.S. Department of Agriculture. *Composition of Dairy and Egg Products: Raw-Processed-Prepared.* 1976.

Notes

Notes

Notes

Notes

Notes

Notes

Notes